# Optical Coherence Tomography
## A Clinical Atlas of Retinal Images

Darrin A. Landry, CRA, OCT-C

*Bryson Taylor Publishing*

Publisher: **Bryson Taylor Publishing**

Author: **Darrin A. Landry, CRA, OCT-C**

Cover Design and Layout: **Donna Berger**
Edited by: **Bryson Taylor Publishing**

ISBN   978-0-9841934-4-8
Library of Congress Control Number 2010918505

Images provided by:
Darrin A. Landry
Eyecare Medical Group, Portland, Maine
David Cimino, CRA
Allison Schmidt, CRA
Heidelberg Engineering
Ray Northway
Carl Zeiss Meditec
Optovue Inc.
Tim Bennett, CRA, FOPS

First Printing January 2011
Printed in the United States of America

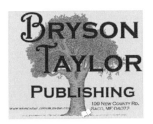

*Bryson Taylor Publishing*
199 New County Road
Saco ME 04072
207-838-2146
www.brysontaylorpublishing.com

**Disclaimer:** All diagnosis' printed or inferred in this book were made by the ophthalmologists in charge of that particular patient's care, and not by the author.

# Table of Contents

*"Light is time thinking about itself."*
Octavio Paz

# I.   Introduction

Optical coherence tomography (OCT) is one of the most commonly used imaging devices in ophthalmic practices. It is capable of generating cross-sectional views of the retina and provides qualitative as well as quantitative data of retinal pathologies.[1]

In this book, we will try to illustrate various common (and some not so common) retinal disease pathologies as presented on OCT, with images from different OCT systems. As OCT technology is an ever-changing field, the information provided in this book is presented using the most recent technology and information at the time of publication.

When OCT was commercially introduced in 1995, ophthalmic practice was dramatically altered. Here was an instrument that allowed for cross sectional imaging of retinal layers, which up to this point could not be done without surgical biopsy and microscopic examination. Using a super luminescent diode light source of 800nm that is capable of axial resolution of about 10 microns and axial depth of 2mm, the most common Time Domain system on the market is the Stratus OCT (Carl Zeiss Meditec, Dublin, CA). [2] Since that time, many other companies have come forward with Fourier, or Spectral Domain technology, all of which are essentially a variation on a theme. Spectral Domain OCT technology uses a stationary spectrometer, which eliminates the need for a moving reference mirror that the Time Domain OCT systems use. This allows for faster acquisition of images (over 20,000 A scans per second) [3] versus the 400 A scans per second from the Stratus OCT [4] and increased sensitivity, resulting in improved image quality. Spectral Domain OCT systems offer better axial resolution of 5 microns, versus the Stratus OCT resolution of 2 microns. Spectral domain OCT also offers image stacking which can be processed to produce 3-dimensional representations of retinal structures as well as 3-dimensional eye mapping. There are currently eight manufacturers of Spectral Domain OCT [5] with more certainly to join the market. Like fundus cameras, most OCT systems operate and produce images that are recognizable, with the differences being in database management, image manipulation, and image output. With this new wealth of information, physicians can not only make better-informed clinical decisions, but also can now better understand the pathophysiology of retinal diseases, and can visualize and quantify change within the retinal layers. OCT retinal thickness measurements have been, and continue to be used for many clinical trials related to retinal vascular diseases.

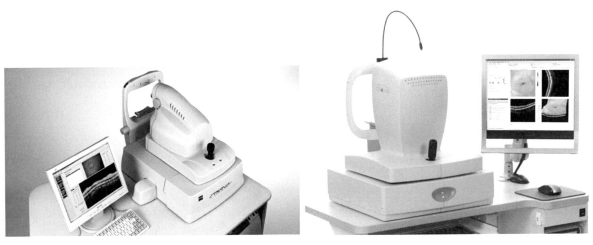

**Zeiss Stratus**                    **Optovue RTVueOCT**

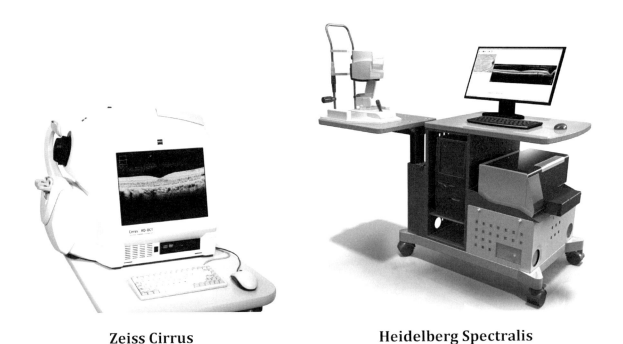

**Zeiss Cirrus**                    **Heidelberg Spectralis**

**Some examples of OCT systems available in today's market**

With new technology comes responsibility. OCT manufacturers are constantly making systems that are more user-friendly, both in hardware and software. What has not changed is the need for the OCT operator to understand retinal disease pathology, ocular anatomy, and basic recognition of OCT findings, to say nothing about knowing how the OCT system operates. Let us tackle these issues one at a time.

The technician, or imager, who operates the OCT, must understand how retinal disease processes may affect a patient's vision. OCT systems, for the most part, rely on a patient's subjective fixation for alignment of the scan. Without physically moving the scan line, an operator relies on the system to scan directly through the fixation target, regardless of where the patient is actually fixating. In diseases that may affect central fixation, such as macular holes or macular degeneration, the patient may not be able to fixate on a central target. The patient may report that they can see the fixation light, but unbeknownst to them they may actually be fixating with an area of the macula that is not affected by visual defect, and which may fall outside the fovea. This is a common problem, and may result in a scan not crossing the central fovea. An operator that understands retinal disease should be able to recognize this, and remedy this by instructing the patient to continue to subjectively fixate centrally. The operator can then move the scan, using the scan results and visualization of the retinal anatomy to scan properly through the fovea. OCT is a dynamic test, and ideally should be treated as thus. Unfortunately, the physician would not be able to stand over the shoulder of the imager, dictating where the scan should be placed. Instead, the responsibility of a quality scan that illustrates the correct scan placement lies solely with the imager.

This brings us to the second point; technicians must have a working knowledge and recognition of ocular, more specifically retinal, anatomy. This greatly enhances the success of an OCT scan. A majority of the OCT scans are performed through the fovea, and it is critical that the technician can recognize the location of the fovea, especially when scanning the aforementioned patients who may not be able to fixate properly. When it is also necessary to scan outside the fovea, the technician needs to be able to recognize where the scan line needs to be placed.

Another area that a majority of technicians may not be strong in is OCT pattern recognition. This is not to say that technicians should be able to diagnose findings on an OCT, but they should be able to recognize and identify basic layers of the retina represented on an OCT scan, as well as be able to differentiate dense structures, such as drusen, versus echo-lucent areas, such as fluid. This will enhance the technician's OCT skills by helping them to recognize a normal OCT scan versus an abnormal scan, and help them to identify artifacts that may be caused by patient, OCT system or operator error.

Having a basic understanding of how an OCT system works also helps the technician to understand how anatomy and disease pathology is represented on the OCT scan. OCT generates a cross sectional image of the retina by measuring the light echo time delay and intensity of the backscattered light, using an infrared wavelength of light at 800-nm. [6] The resulting image mimics a pathology cross section of the retinal tissue. In tissue that absorb light or scatter light greater, the resulting light decreases with depth.

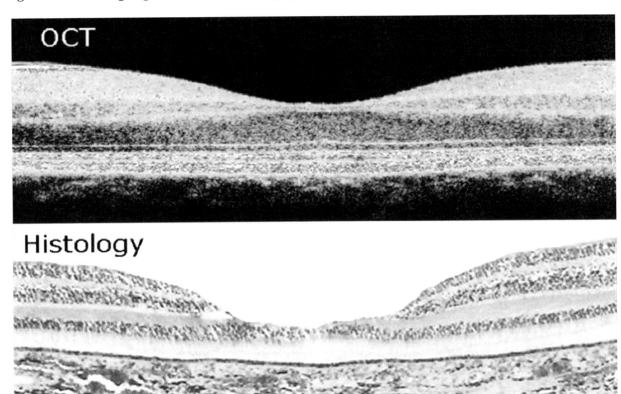

This technology is similar to ultrasound, but uses light waves instead of sound waves. [7]

This knowledge will also be useful for the technician to recognize and remedy artifacts they may encounter as well. As with any imaging modality, communication between the ordering physician and the technician is crucial.

The absolute keys to a successful OCT practice is proper initial scan placement and repeatability of that scan. If a patient is being followed for a specific retinal disease, such as wet macular degeneration, proper scan placement at baseline is only half of what is necessary. Subsequent scans must be placed in the same exact location in order to recognize change from the baseline scan. More recent OCT systems have software that allows the user to request that a scan be placed in the exact location as a previous scan. Using anatomical landmarks, the software does just that. Older systems, specifically Time Domain technology, may not have this function, and therefore the technician must use anatomical landmarks to repeat the line scan. This is where proper training is important. After all, OCT scanning should be a dynamic, not static testing device. Accepting the first scan produced by the system is not acceptable- the operator, armed with knowledge of disease pathology, ocular anatomy, and a basic understanding of how the OCT system works will be able to produce quality, repeatable scans that are clinically viable.

The physician places an immense amount of responsibility in the hands of the technician. The image produced will, in many cases, determine the diagnosis and may dictate clinical treatment.

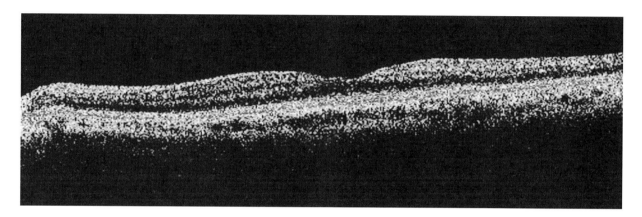

**Normal retina on Time Domain OCT**

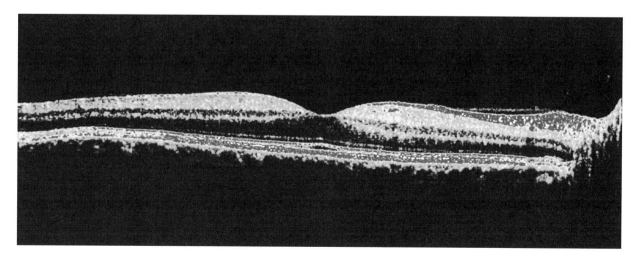

**Normal retina in color on Spectral Domain OCT**

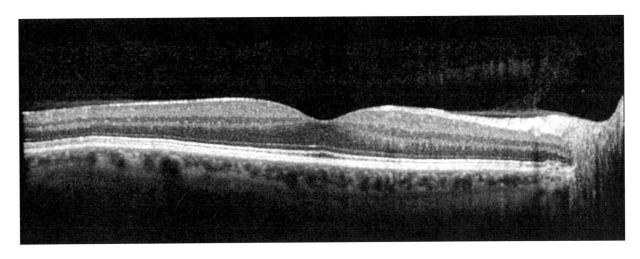

**Normal retina in black and white on Spectral Domain**

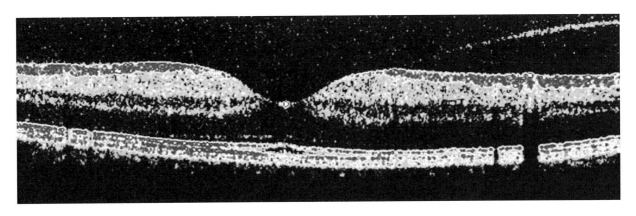

**Normal bright foveal reflex**

Time Domain OCT software assigns false color to tissue depending on density, therefore Time Domain OCT is typically presented in color. Spectral Domain offers the option of color or black and white. Because the color assigned to layers of the retina is so bright, and tissue is more defined on Spectral Domain OCT, in many cases the tissue layer delineation may be obscured by the brightness of the colors. In this book you will see examples of both color and black and white.

# II.    Descriptive Interpretation of OCT

As mentioned previously, OCT is a standard clinical imaging tool that when performed properly can provide invaluable clinical information for the physician. In order to perform a proper scan, the technician must understand how OCT works, be able to identify ocular anatomy, and understand retinal pathophysiologic disease process. All of these are key to providing true information to the clinician and will assist in better clinical and treatment decisions. One of the tools a technician should employ is the ability to descriptively interpret an OCT scan. Technicians are not responsible for diagnosing disease based on OCT, but can better their technique by understanding how to descriptively interpret the scan.

Reviewing one's work has always been a requisite for imagers, and this certainly holds true with OCT. The clinician is basing diagnosis and treatment plans on the print of the scan from the technician (although computer based review is becoming more common). Before the clinician receives the image, the technician needs to review his or her work to ensure a proper scan was obtained. Being able to recognize how retinal disease manifests on an OCT is one of the best ways to make certain a scan is accurate.

Because OCT assigns false colors (or, in the case of black and white- shades of gray) according to the density of tissue, OCT is interpreted by levels of density. In the case of black and white, borders of retinal layers may be easier to distinguish without the blooming effect that false color may provide. Dense tissue has a higher reflectivity, and will be illustrated in color as red or white. Less dense tissue, such as neurosensory retina, is represented as yellow or green, and even less dense tissue and fluid is represented as black. On black and white images, levels of gray are used to represent density of tissue. The brighter the intensity of gray, the denser the tissue. Understanding and recognizing the layers of the retina seen on OCT will help the imager to distinguish pathology and recognize artifacts and true disease.

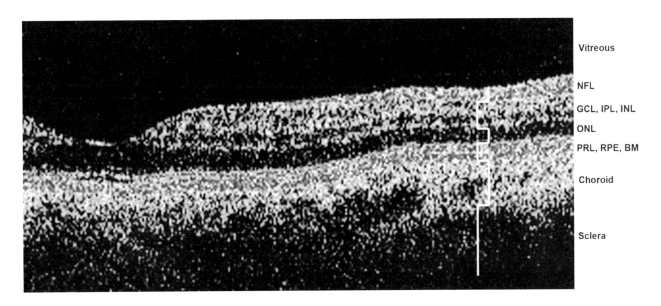

**3a. Layers of the retina as seen on Time Domain OCT**

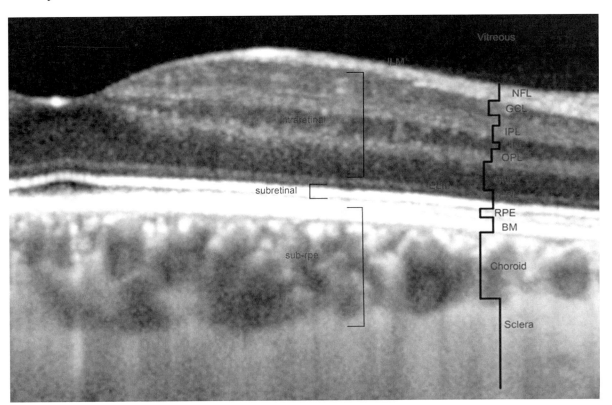

**3b. Layers of the retina as seen on Spectral Domain OCT**

(**NFL**- nerve fiber layer, **GCL**- ganglion cell layer, **IPL**- inner plexiform layer, **INL**- inner nuclear layer, **ONL**- outer nuclear layer, **PRL**- photoreceptor cell layer, **RPE**- retinal pigment epithelium, **BM**- Bruch's membrane)

Knowing all layers of the retina is probably not necessary when it comes to descriptive interpretation. Most retinal diseases affect either the sub-RPE space, sub retinal space (which lies above the RPE and below the interface of the segments of the photoreceptor layer), or intraretinal (defined by the space above the interface of the photoreceptor layer and below the RNFL), the anterior retina or the vitreoretinal interface.

Understanding a patient's retinal disease pathology is extremely helpful for the imager. A patient who has macular disease, such as macular degeneration or a macular hole, may not be able to fixate properly. Most OCT devices rely on a subjective fixation to scan through. If the patient does not fixate centrally, due to a central visual defect, the OCT may scan parafoveally, or outside the pathologic fovea. The simple fix is to have the patient fixate subjectively, and then physically move the scan to identify the fovea. *(Images 1 and 2)* In order to execute this properly, the technician must be able to recognize retinal anatomy. This particular issue will be revisited as it pertains to specific retinal disease throughout this book.

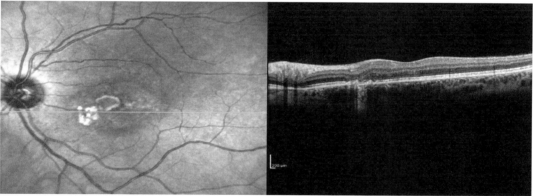

**1. Spectral Domain image scanned below the fovea, through subjective fixation**

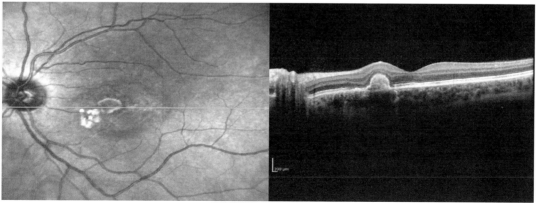

**2. Spectral Domain image scanned through the fovea, after the user moved the scan**

OCT systems are very susceptible to eye movement, as well as outside interference as demonstrated in the examples below.

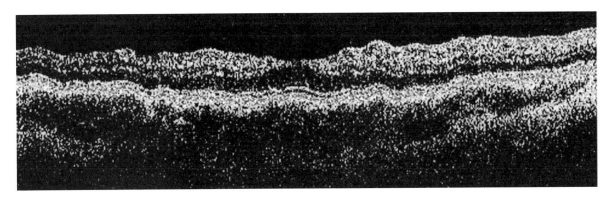

**Building HVAC system under the floor in the OCT room can cause movement artifact. Note the "ripple effect" throughout the retinal layers**

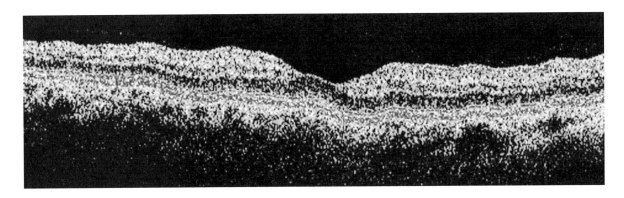

**Patient with nystagmus**

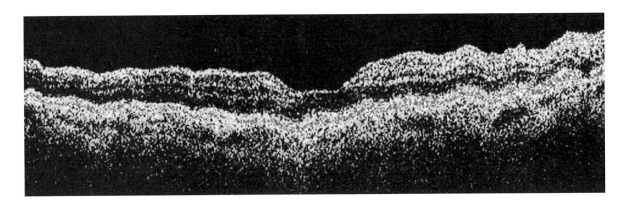

**Patient with head tremor**

## Moving the Scan

To combat patient eye movement, and to ensure that subsequent scans are in the same exact placement as original scans, some Spectral Domain systems have software that "track" eye movement, using retinal blood vessel patterns as landmarks to place the line scan in the same location as previously designated by the user. The system does not interpret pathology, so if an initial scan is performed in the wrong area, subsequent scans will produce the same wrong image.

In the case of Time Domain OCT, it is up to the operator to recognize anatomy and move the scan appropriately. This does introduce user error possibilities, but needs to be performed if the patient is not properly fixating. By moving the mouse arrow onto the screen and holding the mouse button, the operator can move the scan until it is lined up in the right area. This can be done with both line scans and macular thickness radial scans.

In the following example, note that the original scan was properly placed through the fovea, and set as a reference. The second image shows the same patient but now fixating nasally. The software recognizes the retinal blood vessels from the previously referenced scan and, despite eccentric fixation, scans the exact same location.

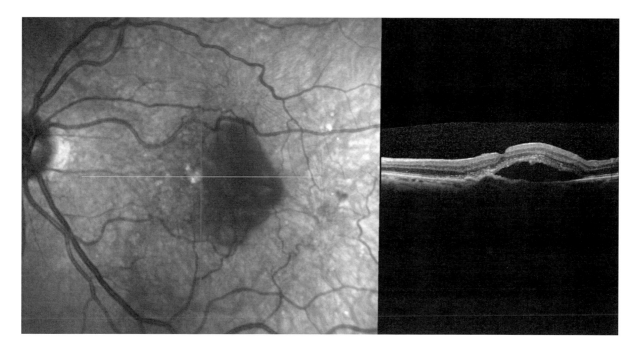

**Original scan**

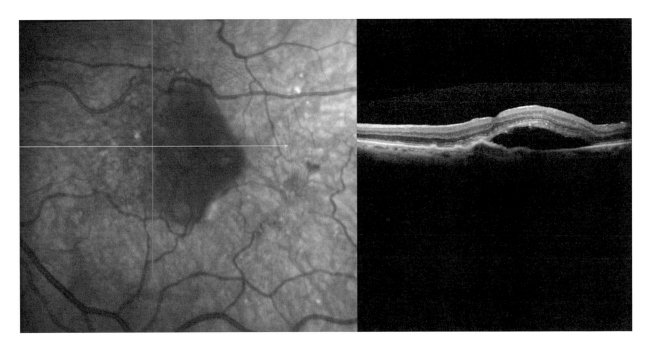

**Follow up scan. Note the fundus image has moved, but the scan is in the same axis**

### Capturing and Analyzing Images

OCT imaging is a two-step process, and in the case of Time Domain OCT, the steps are separately executed by the imager. Most Spectral Domain OCT systems process the steps automatically. The first is to properly scan the retina. The second is to choose the proper protocol algorithm in which to process the image through. Volumetric OCT, which will be discussed next, is also a two-step process, with a number of different analysis algorithms that reflect the volumetric measurement of an area of retina, either in false color display or numerically. On the following page is an example of an RPE detachment captured on Time Domain OCT with a single line scan. Note the raw scan; that is, the scan imaged prior to being processed through the analysis protocol. What follows are the different choices of analysis protocols on the Stratus system (Carl Zeiss Meditec, Dublin, CA). There is no set protocol for line scans, it is up to the particular physician to view the raw image processed and determine which analysis protocol provides the most accurate image.

**Analysis protocols for line scan on Time Domain OCT**

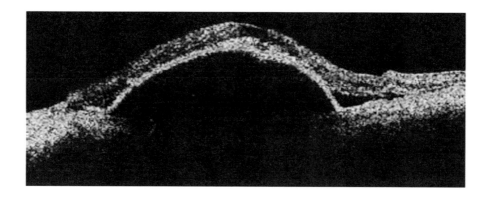

Raw image

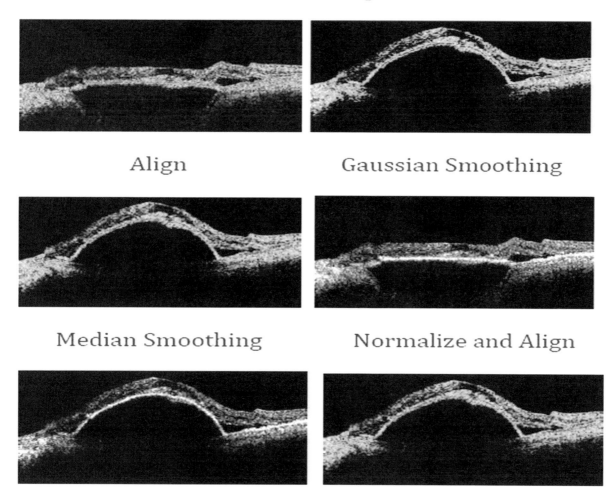

Align  Gaussian Smoothing

Median Smoothing  Normalize and Align

Normalize  Proportional

# III. Volumetric OCT

Volumetric OCT is a scan and analysis protocol that is particularly useful for following progression or regression of intraretinal fluid as well as sub retinal fluid. With the algorithm used in the Stratus, or Time Domain system, the measurement for volume is taken from a radial scan, either a fast macular thickness or macular thickness scan. It is important to note that the Stratus system uses segmentation boundary lines that measure the thickness of the retina from the ILM (internal limiting membrane, which is the most anterior layer of the retina) to the anterior aspect of the RPE, therefore any sub-RPE fluid is not taken into account when volumetric analysis is performed. This is an issue that needs to be recognized by the imager and interpreter of the images prior to making a clinical decision based on volumetric OCT. Knowing this, the imager and interpreter must make a decision as to initial and follow up scans performed on these patients. A volumetric OCT is very helpful to establish a baseline and to "see the big picture", but should be used with caution in follow up of cases of sub-RPE fluid. Disease pathologies that manifest themselves with intraretinal fluid, such as cystoid macular edema, diabetic macular edema, vein occlusions, etc., present as excellent subjects for baseline and follow up volumetric OCT. Time Domain and most Spectral Domain OCT systems offer a change analysis protocol, which will determine the difference in volume from one scan to another, and illustrate the difference in both color and numeric values.

In the Time Domain OCT images that follow, note that the processed scan flattens the elevation of the RPE and the resulting volumetric measurements indicates a normal foveal depression, as mentioned previously. Therefore, in the case of sub-RPE fluid, volumetric measurements on Time Domain OCT should be flagged or noted. This is a case where a qualitative line scan is much more useful than a quantitative volumetric scan.

Here is the raw scan of a PED:

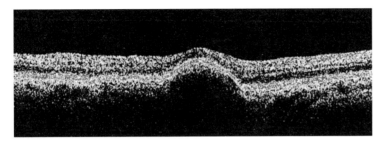

The volumetric analysis:

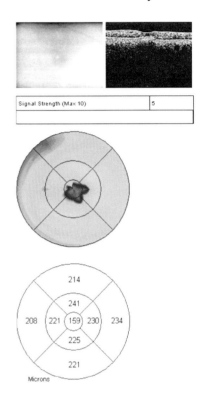

Here is the resulting analysis(note the measurement lines at the ILM and RPE):

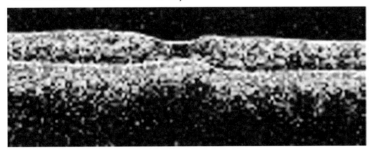

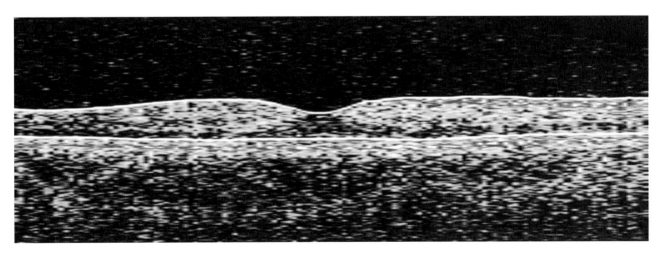

Note that the boundary lines (in white) are at the level of the ILM and the anterior aspect of the retinal pigment epithelium

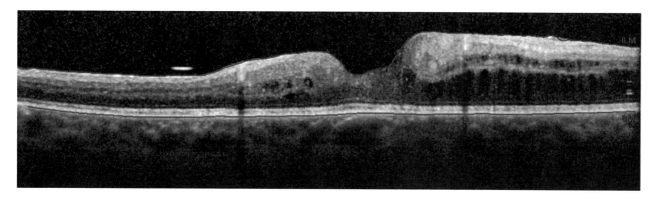

**In spectral domain, the boundary lines (in red) are at the ILM and Bruch's Membrane**

In the cases of sub-RPE fluid, a qualitative line scan on the Stratus system is more accurate than a quantitative volumetric scan. An example of this, using a 7mm line scan with a 7-degree offset, allows a scan to be "anchored" at the midline of the temporal edge of the optic nerve head, and the 7 degree offset will natural cross the fovea in most cases. This can then be repeated on subsequent scans. The steps for creating this scan are as follows:

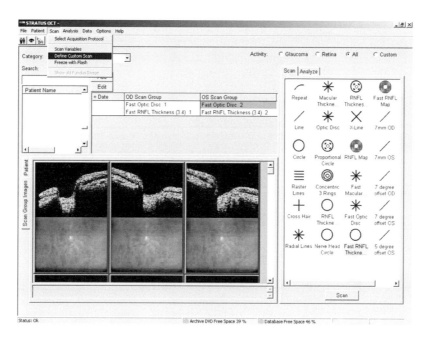

1. Click on *Scan*, then *Define Custom Scan*

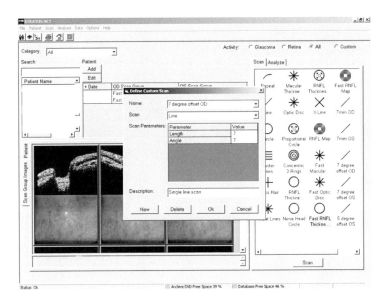

2. Fill in the open window with the above information for the right eye (Name, Scan, Length and Angle) note the angle is set at 7

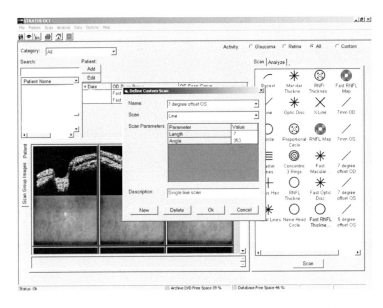

3. Repeat the same steps for the left eye, name the scan 7 degree offset OS (note the angle is set at 353)

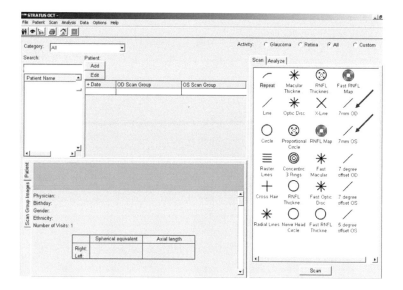

4. Note the new scans are now in the scan protocol window

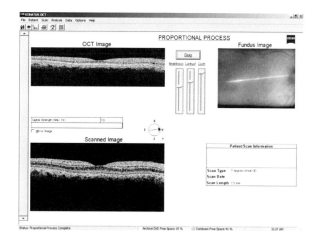

**7mm offset line scan OD**

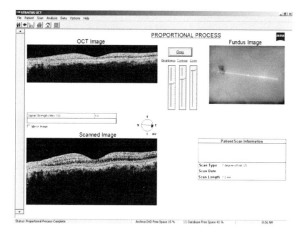

**7mm offset line scan OS**

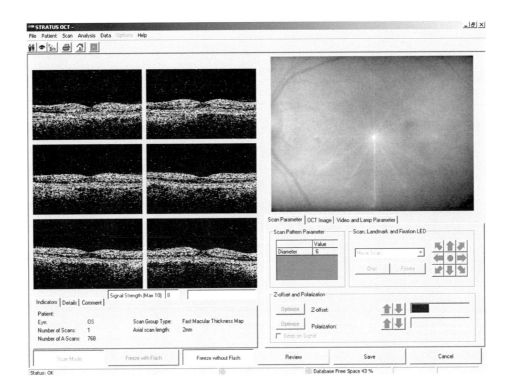

## Radial scans used in Fast Macular scan on Time Domain OCT

Time Domain OCT uses multiple scans, typically in a radial pattern, to produce a measurement of volume in the area scanned. The most common scans used for this is the Macular Thickness, or Fast Macular Thickness Map. The difference between them is the amount of "A" scans, or data points used to create the measurement. The Fast Macular Map uses 128, whereas the Macular Thickness Map uses 512, producing a much better "resolution" image of the retina.

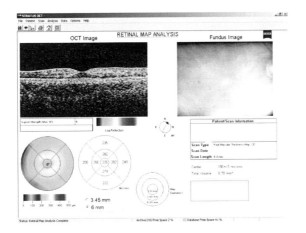

**Fast macular thickness map**

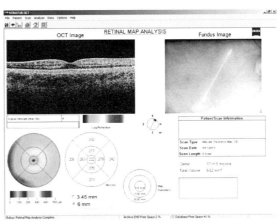

**Macular thickness map**

14

Volumetric OCT is particularly useful for following the amount of volumetric change in retinal tissue on subsequent visits, and especially after treatment of intraretinal fluid. The software will not only show false color and numerical volumetric measurements, but can also display change analysis between images, represented in both color and numeric values. Normal foveal thickness is approximately 120-150 microns in younger adults and 175-220 microns in older adults 8

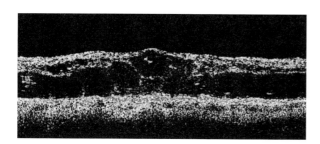 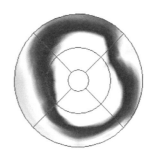

**Pre treatment**

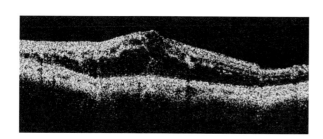 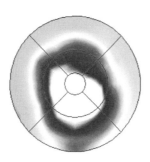

**One treatment session**

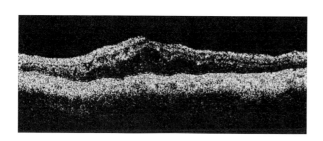 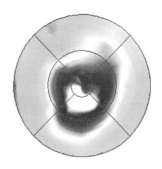

**Second treatment session**

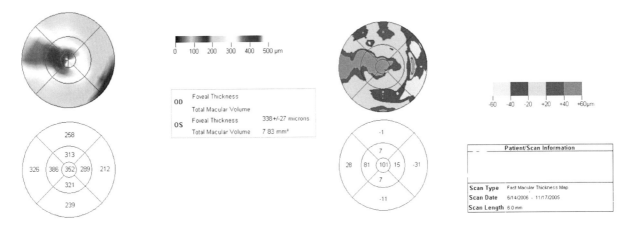

**Pre treatment**                                          **Post treatment change analysis**

Spectral Domain OCT uses many more data points than Time Domain to produce a volumetric measurement, and scans can either be in a radial or linear pattern.

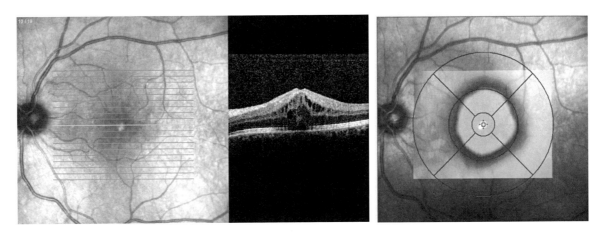

**Raster scan (on the left), which uses a linear pattern of scans either horizontally or vertically, produces a color display (on the right) representing retinal tissue volume**

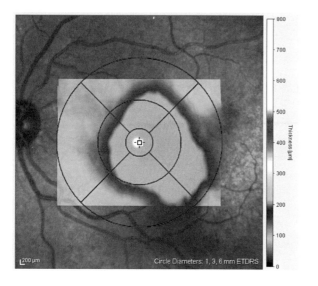

**Mac edema pre treatment volumetric OCT**     **Post treatment volumetric OCT**

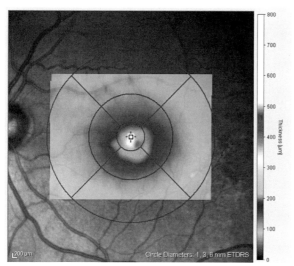

**Macular edema pre treatment**

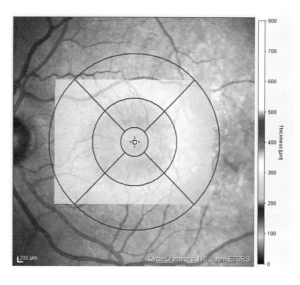

**Post treatment**

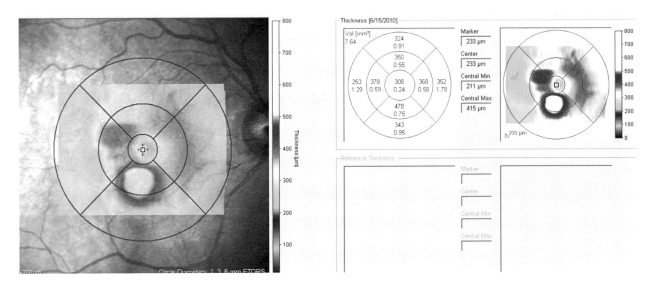

**Volumetric OCT of an inferior RPE detachment**

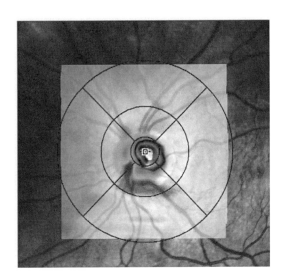

**Normal volumetric OCT of optic nerve head**

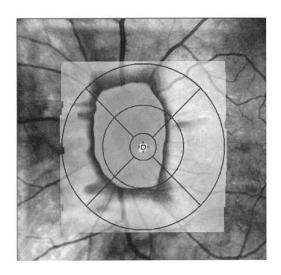

**Volumetric OCT of optic nerve head with papilledema**

# IV.   Atlas of Images

The retina is a complex, multilayer structure that is responsible for receiving light and converting it to neural impulses, which are interpreted by the brain. The central area of the retina, which is where the concentration of ganglion cells are located, is called the macula. It is about 5.5mm in diameter, and is within the superior and inferior vascular arcades. The anatomic fovea, which is a central depression in the center of the macula, is only about 1.5mm in diameter, approximately the same size as the optic disc. The anatomic foveola is the central depression that is illustrated on OCT and is about 350 microns in diameter [9]

The best and most productive way to describe OCT findings is to break the anatomy up into 4 sections from anterior to posterior: The vitreous, intraretinal, sub-retinal and sub RPE, or choroidal.

## A. Vitreous

The vitreous is the clear, egg white consistency fluid that fills the back of the eye. It is made up of 99% water and accounts for 80% of the total volume of the globe. The vitreous is attached to the retina, and eventually detaches from the retina in most patients, due to the breakdown of vitreous due to aging. [10] Vitreous traction is a pathology that was never able to be imaged before OCT. Certainly, the effects of vitreous traction, such as edema and holes, were evident on both ophthalmoscopy and even fluorescein angiography, but the actual mechanical traction that caused these issues was not evident. In some cases, imaging vitreous traction and treating surgically before it causes other problems may help stem severe vision problems, such as macular holes, detachments, or vitreous hemorrhages.

We have chosen to include epiretinal membranes in this section, as they are visualized on OCT at the level above the nerve fiber layer, although the effect of epiretinal membranes can be seen in the layer that is termed "intraretinal". Epiretinal membranes may present as a distinct dense layer above the NFL, and can sometimes be very adherent to the retina, which may give the impression of a normal retina. These membranes may also present as a separate entity, separated from the retina by space between the membrane and the retina. The effect of the traction caused by the membrane can be seen as intraretinal fluid or hemorrhages, caused by vascular leakage and edema. Psuedoholes of the macula may also be present, caused by openings in the membrane overlying the fovea. [11] Epiretinal membranes also have been described as cellophane retinopathy and macular pucker. [12]

## Vitreous Traction

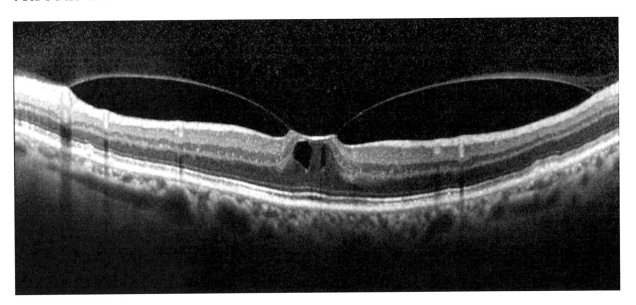

Vitreomacular traction. Note the attachments temporal, nasal, and central. There is also intraretinal edema present due to the mechanical traction

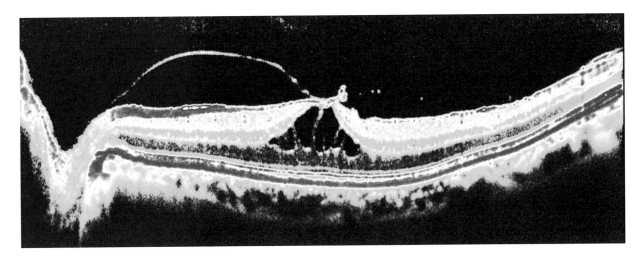

Vitreomacular traction with intraretinal edema

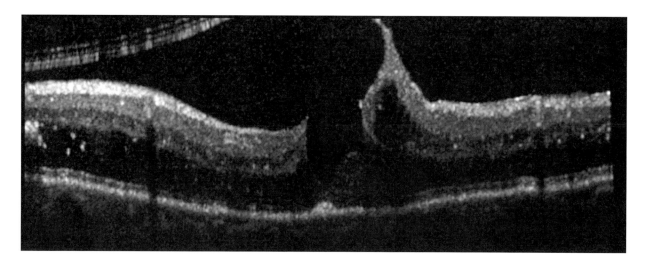

In this case, the vitreous traction has pulled an area of the macula and created a macular hole

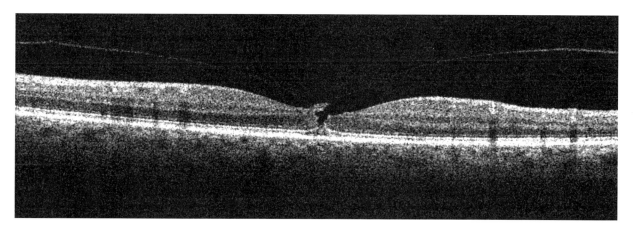

Vitreous traction causing a separation of retinal tissue almost down to the level of RPE

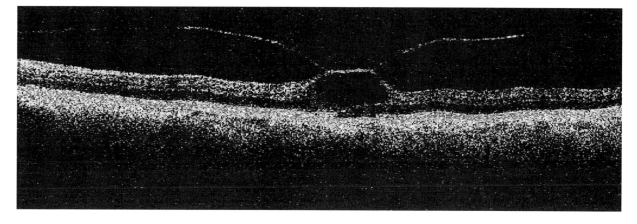

Vitreomacular traction seen on Time Domain OCT. The traction has created a large cyst in the fovea. In some clinical cases, this may be the precursor to a macular hole

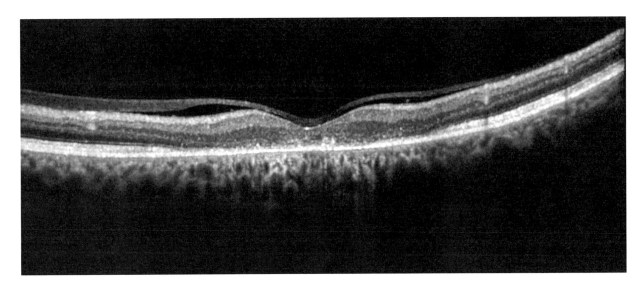

**Partial Posterior Vitreous Detachment**

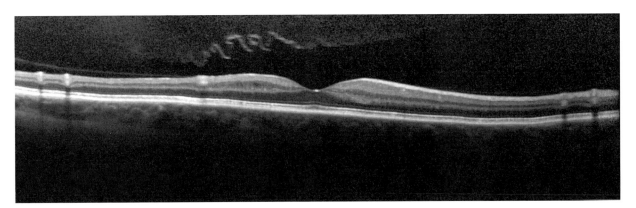

**Partial Posterior Vitreous Detachment**

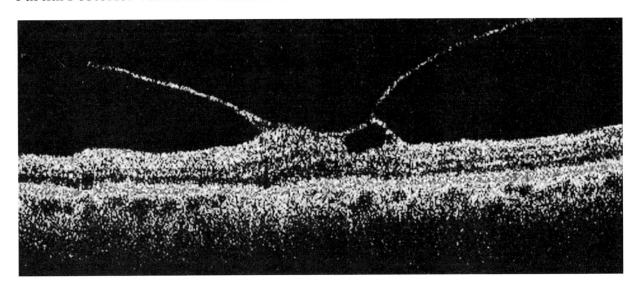

**Vitreomacular traction on Time Domain**

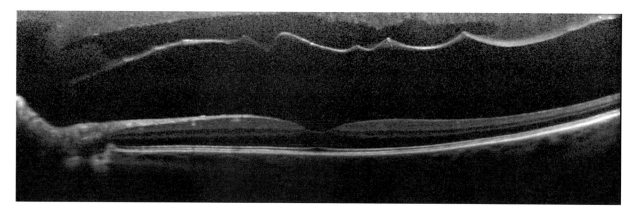

Posterior Vitreous Detachment

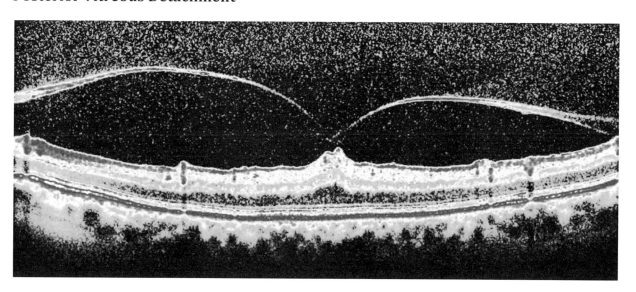

Vitreomacular traction with attachments temporally, nasally and centrally

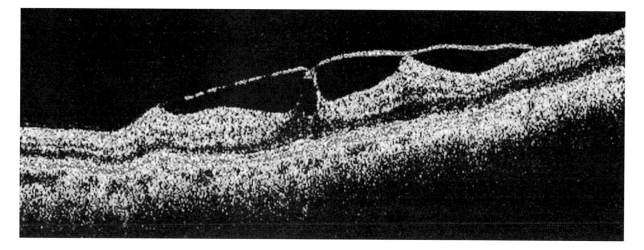

Vitreomacular traction with multiple central attachment points

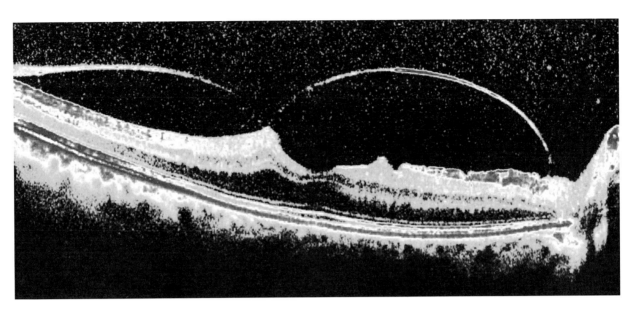

Vitreomacular traction adhered centrally, temporal, and nasal to the fovea

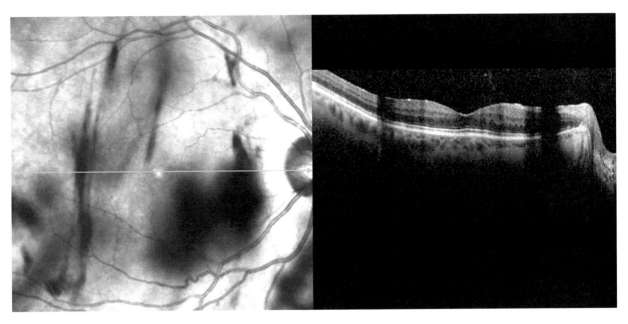

OCT and corresponding fundus image of a patient with a vitreous hemorrhage. As OCT uses light to image, anything that can block light will result in missing data. Note the areas of black shadowing on the OCT that represent missing data due to the light being blocked by the hemorrhage

In many cases of vitreomacular traction, vitreous attachments may not be obviously attached at the retina, but telltale signs of these attachments may be represented by strands of highly reflective vitreous interface. The imager must recognize this finding and move the scan to demonstrate the attached point(s) of the vitreous to macular traction.

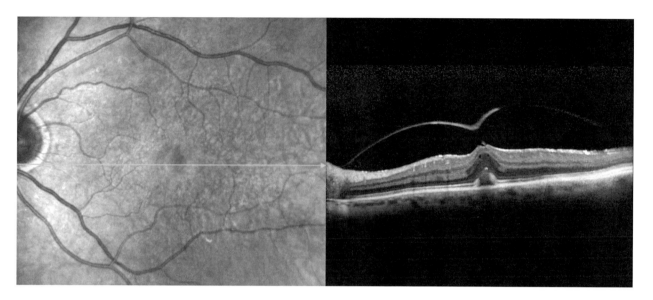

**Macular traction missed, but note the vitreous "pointing" to the fovea**

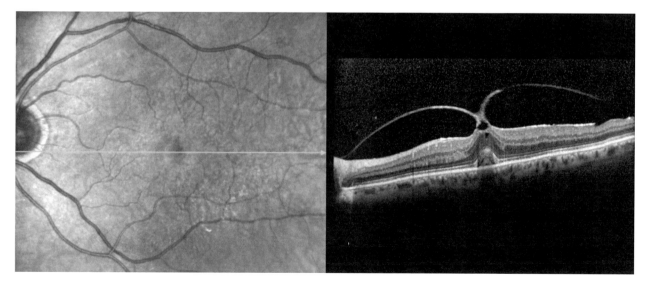

**Same patient after moving the scan, with macular traction now revealed**

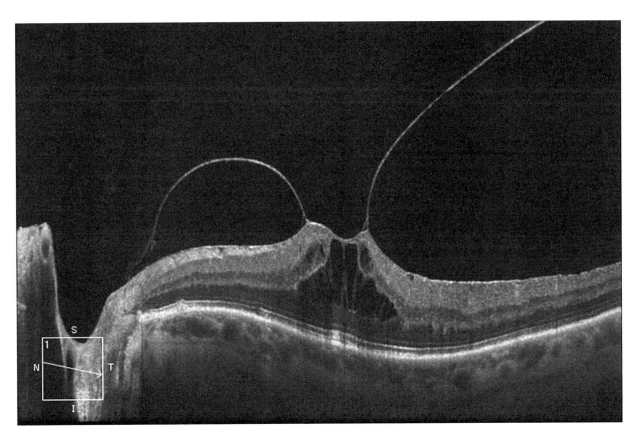

Vitreomacular traction causing cystoid macular edema (CME)

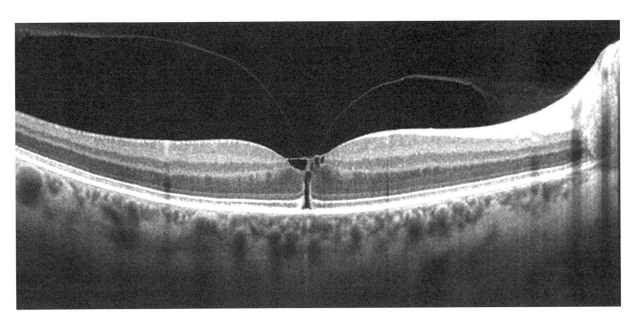

Vitreomacular traction with edema and macular hole

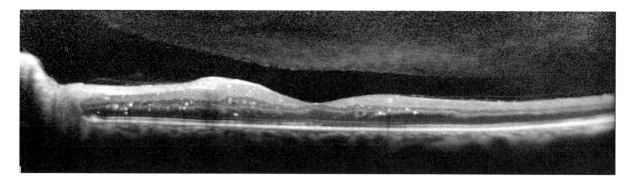

Diabetic patient with red blood cells in the vitreous

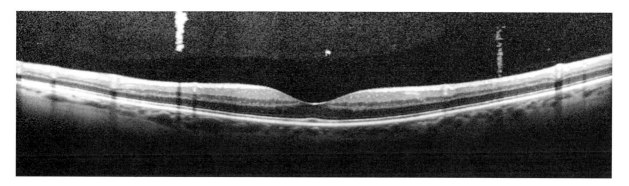

Dense vitreous

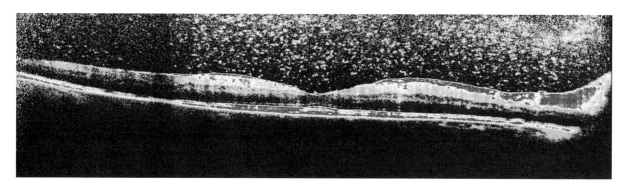

Asteroid Hyalosis

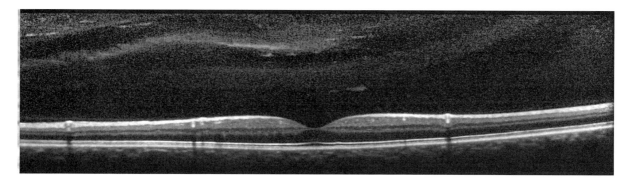

Dense vitreous

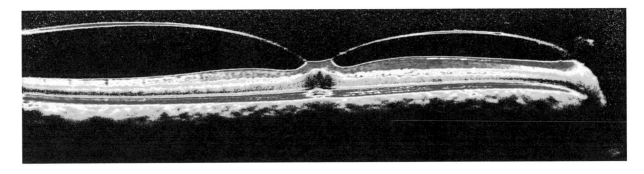

Vitreomacular traction

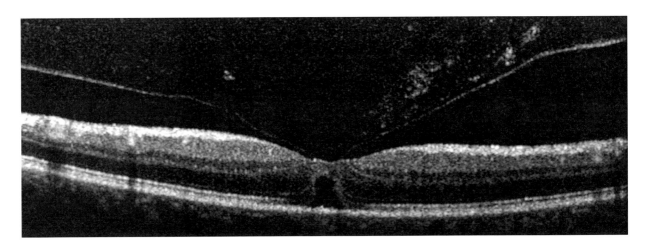

Vitreomacular traction with early macular hole

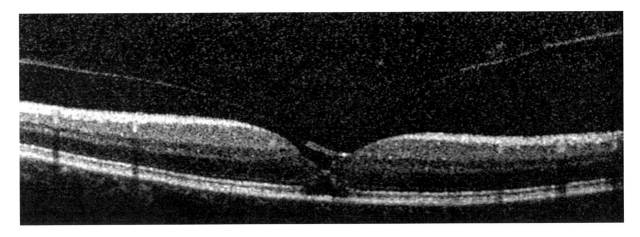

Same patient, now progressed to full thickness macular hole

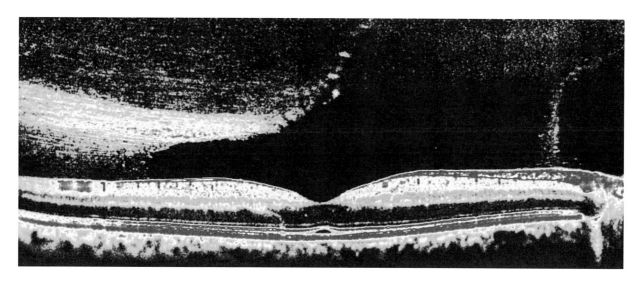

Dense posterior vitreous detachment with some attachments present in the temporal and nasal macular region

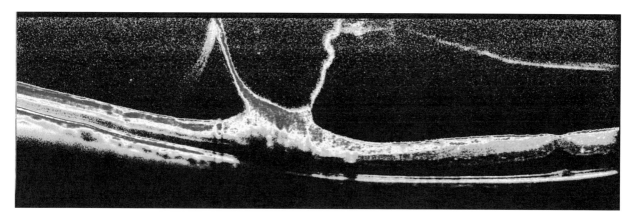

Vitreomacular traction with edematous retina

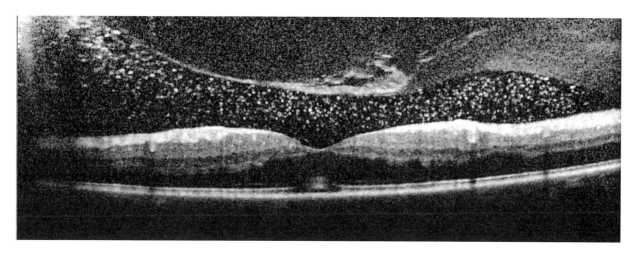

Vitreous hemorrhages can cause dense reflectivity of the OCT light, often times obscuring the retinal detail

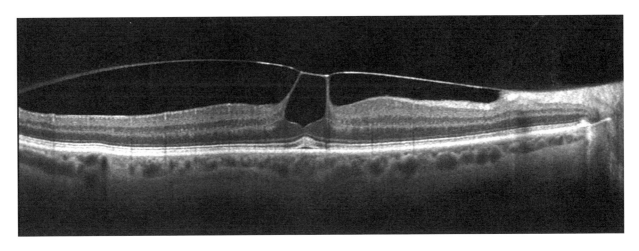

Classic vitreomacular traction, with attachments in the central macula causing a large macular cyst

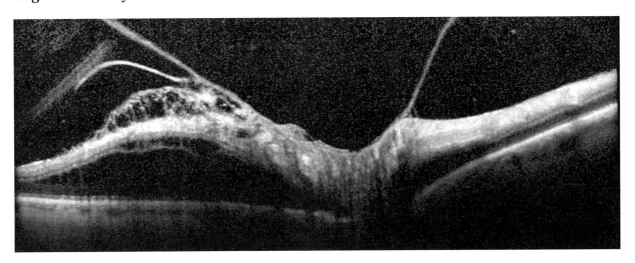

Vitreomacular traction with intraretinal and sub retinal fluid

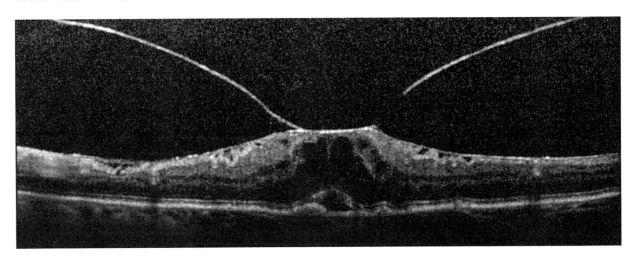

Vitreomacular traction with epiretinal membrane and intraretinal fluid

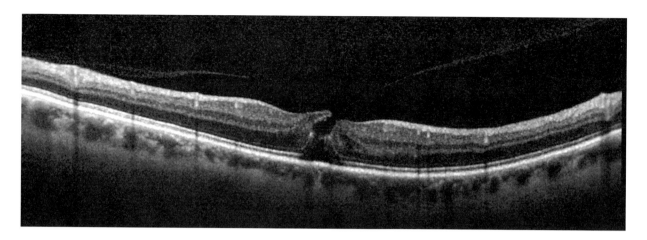

Vitreomacular traction with partial thickness macular hole

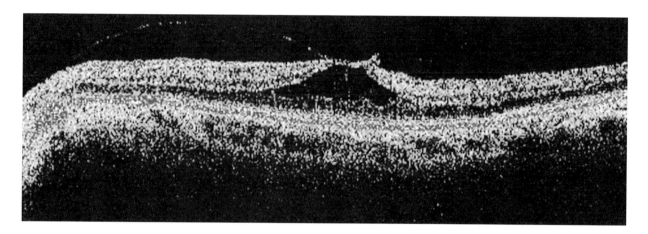

Vitreomacular traction with cystoid macular edema on Time Domain OCT

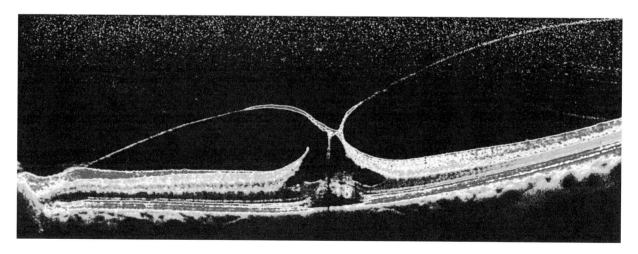

Vitreomacular traction that has pulled macular tissue and created a macular hole

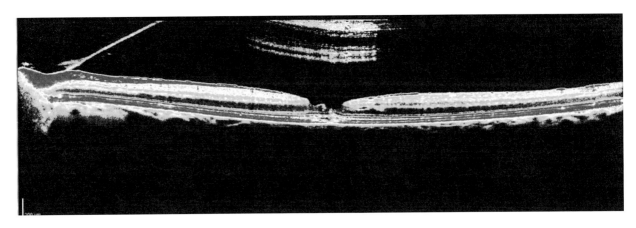

A posterior vitreous detachment with dense reflectivity above the macula. Note the attachment on the nasal side

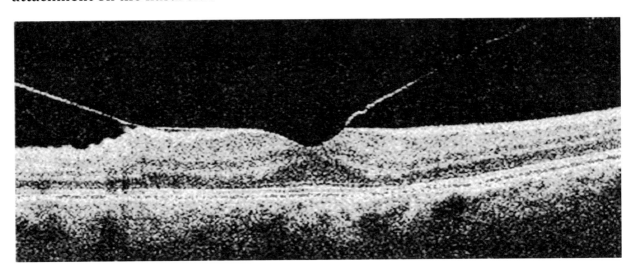

Vitreomacular traction, giving an ERM type appearance on the temporal side

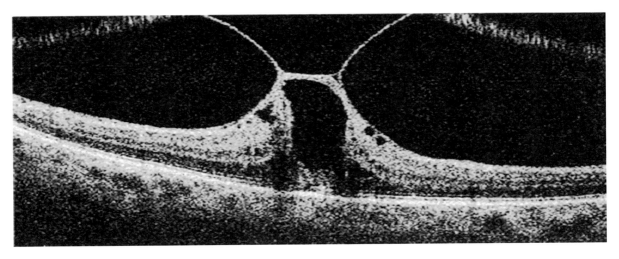

Vitreomacular traction with associated macular edema

## Epiretinal Membranes

Epiretinal membranes are yet another pathology that the OCT is extremely useful for visualizing. Prior to OCT, only the effects of an ERM, such as intraretinal edema, were obvious during clinical exam or fluorescein angiography. The actual mechanical traction was not visible. Patients with symptoms of distortion or blurriness commonly have wrinkling of the internal limiting membrane (ILM) and can have retinal thickening due to edema.[13]

Sometimes epiretinal membranes can cause a loss of foveal depression, making it difficult for the imager to discern the location of the fovea. Oftentimes traction from the membrane can pull the foveal depression up to create a level or straight retinal surface. In these situations, the retinal OCT image will show a pyramid shaped space in the intra retinal layer, with the apex at the point of the previous foveal depression.

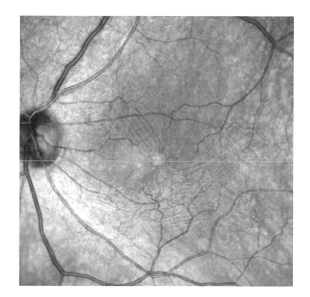 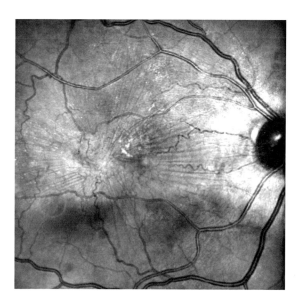

**Fundus images of an epiretinal membrane. Note the striations in the retina**

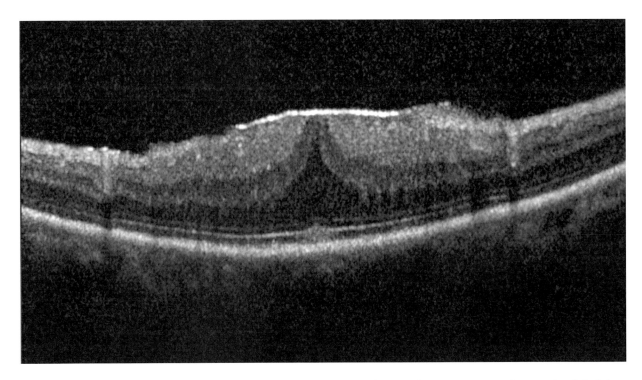

Epiretinal membranes may not have a separation from the retina, and may be highly echogenic, appearing as a separate, denser layer. Also, note the cone shape of the fovea

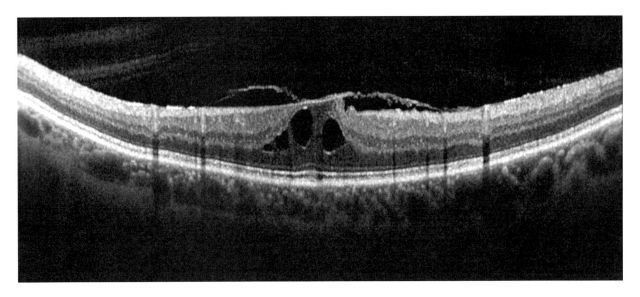

An epiretinal membrane providing traction on the surface of the retina is causing intraretinal fluid. Note the separation of tissue between the membrane and the retina

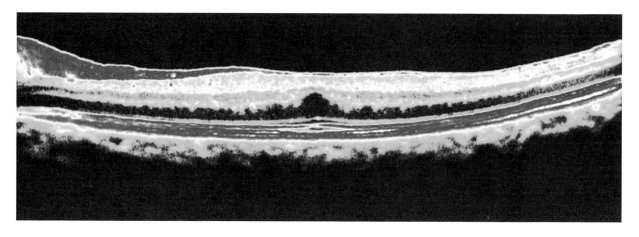

Epiretinal membranes may not appear classic, with a high density reflectivity, but can cause a "tenting" of the fovea. This example shows the classic pyramid space, indicating the fovea

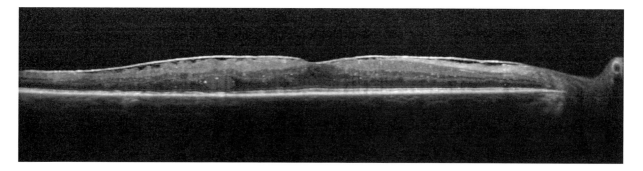

This epiretinal membrane is not causing tractional edema, but can clearly be distinguished from the normal retinal tissue by its separation.

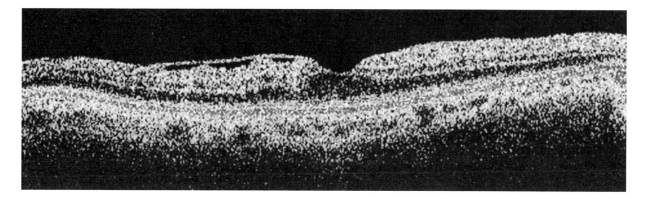

Epiretinal membrane on Time Domain OCT

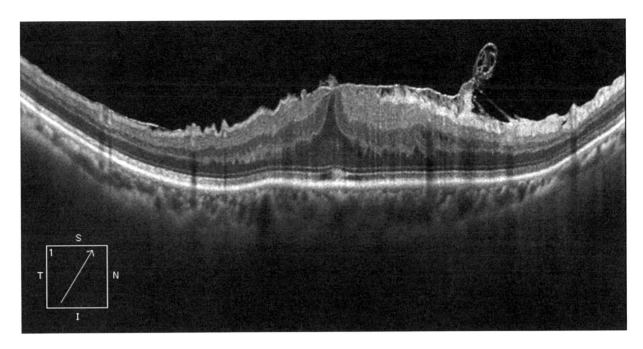

Membranes can sometimes contract or break its traction, which can appear as a "bunching" of tissue on the retinal surface. Also, note the absence of a foveal depression, but the presence of a pyramid shaped space, indicating the fovea

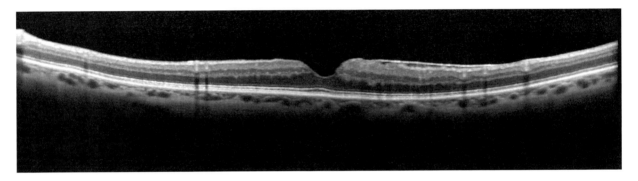

Termed *trace epiretinal membrane*, this is an example of a slight separation between the membrane and the retinal surface, seen temporally, with no edema

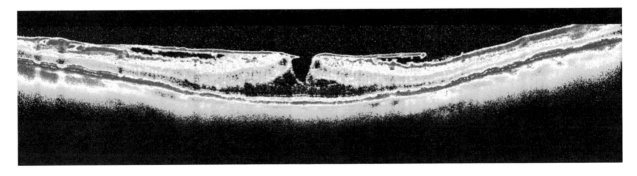

Epiretinal membrane with partial thickness macular hole

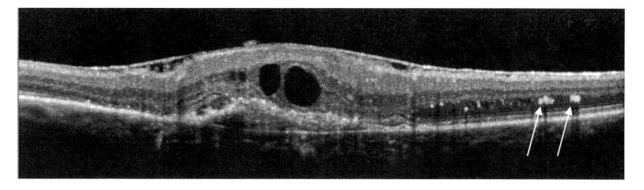

Epiretinal membrane with hard exudates (arrows) unrelated to the ERM

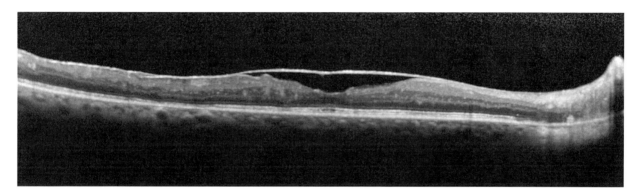

Epiretinal membrane not adhered to the fovea

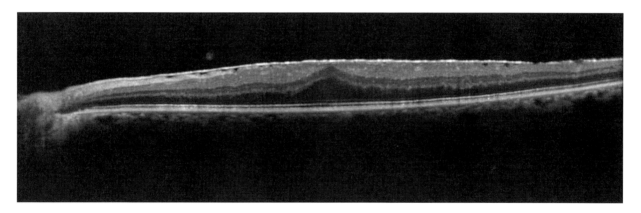

In many cases, the epiretinal membrane can distort the retina and make the fovea difficult to discern. Note the pyramid shape to the previously depressed fovea.

**The following pages are more examples of this type of epiretinal membrane:**

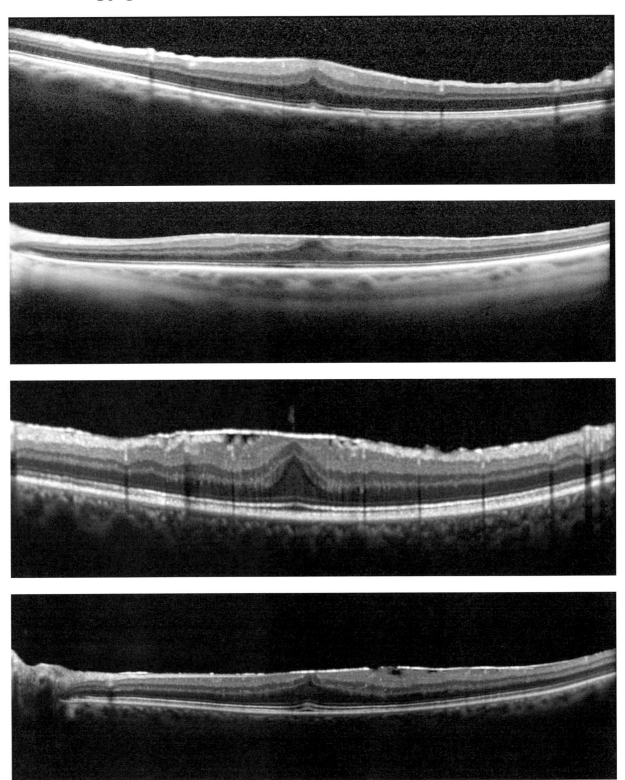

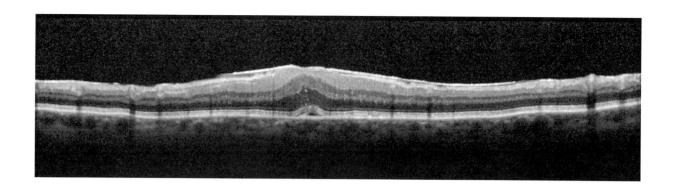

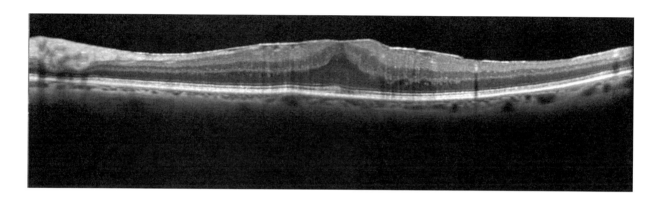

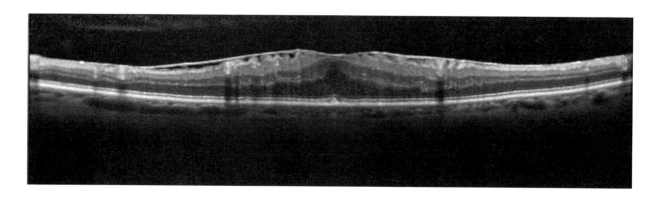

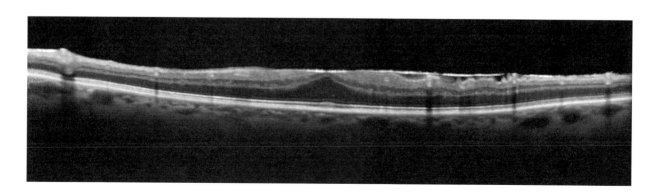

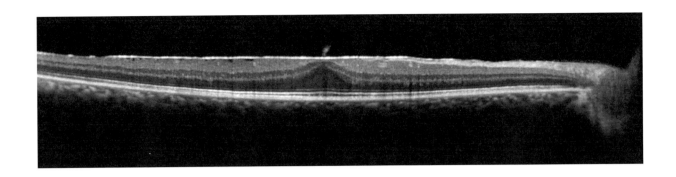

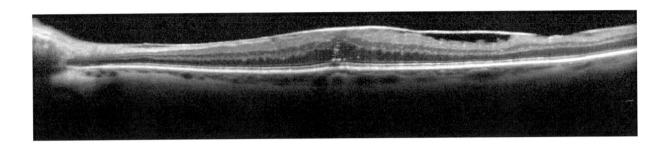

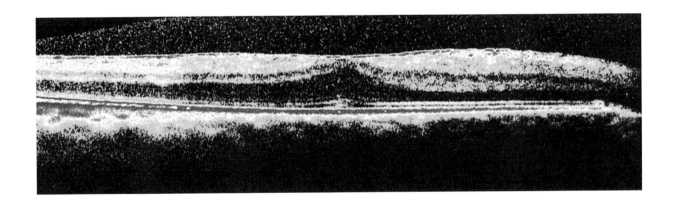

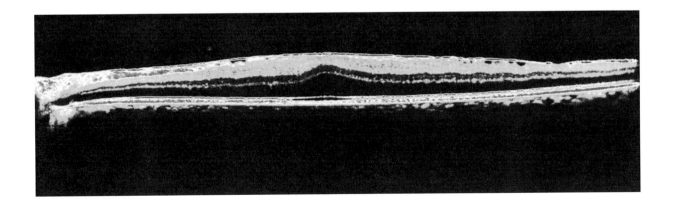

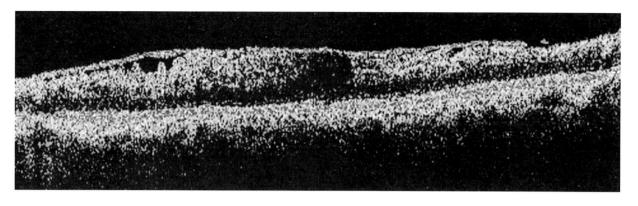

Time Domain OCT of an epiretinal membrane. The fovea is only distinguishable by the shadowed area centrally

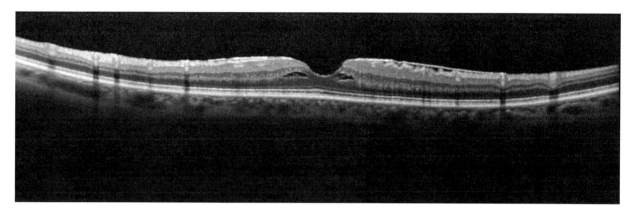

Epiretinal membrane with macular edema, represented by the cystic pockets of fluid on either side of the fovea

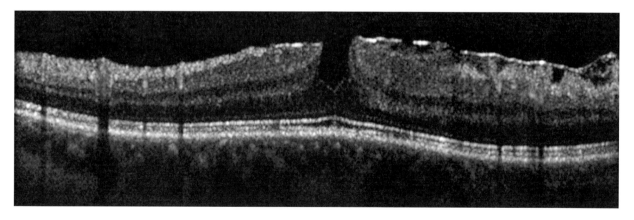

Epiretinal membrane with partial thickness macular hole. Note the high reflectivity of the membrane

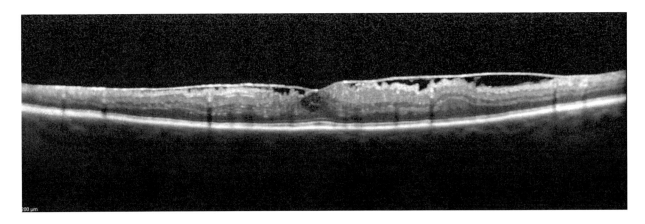

Epiretinal membrane with several attachment points and a foveal cyst

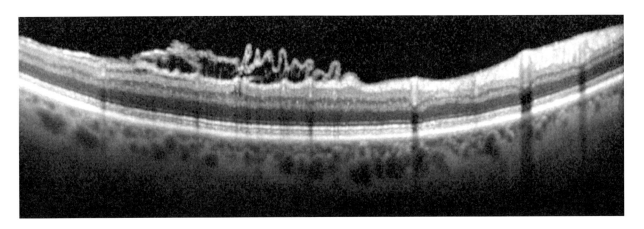

In some cases, the epiretinal membrane can break and coil above the retina. This scan was done outside the fovea, hence the absence of a foveal depression

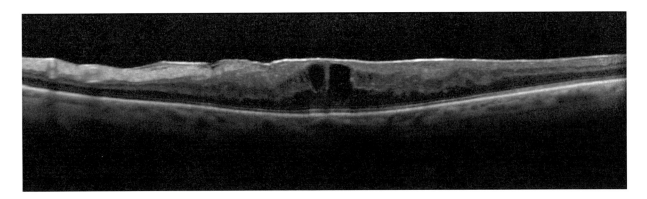

The only indication of an epiretinal membrane in this case is the high reflectivity. Also, note macular edema

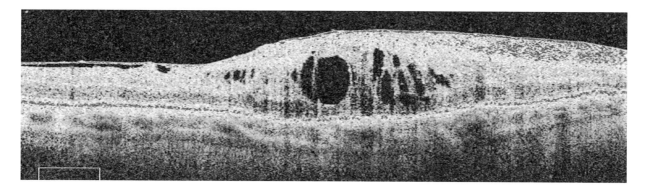

In cases where the membrane has completely distorted the fovea, it is vitally important that the imager scan the entire macular area to discern the foveal location

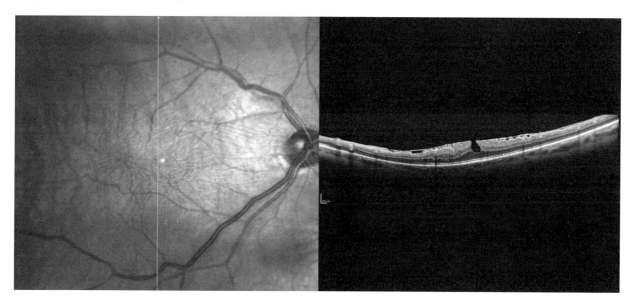

Epiretinal membrane with lamellar hole. Note the striations in the retina on the fundus image

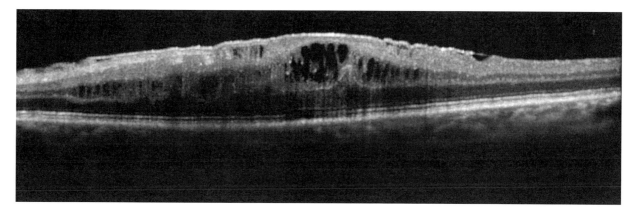

In some cases, it is difficult for the imager and interpreter to see the fovea, and communication between the two is crucial

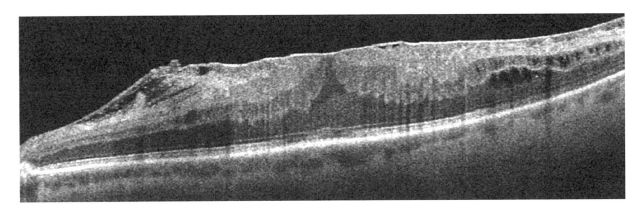

Another example of a flat fovea with the classic pyramid shape beneath it

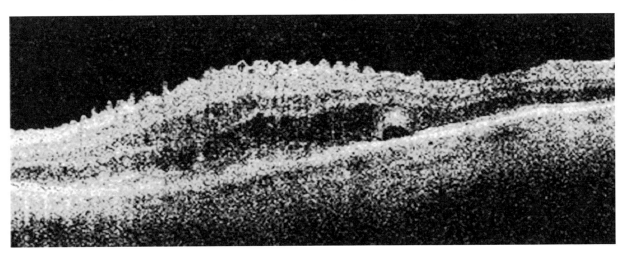

"Bunching" of the retina as a result of an epiretinal membrane outside the fovea

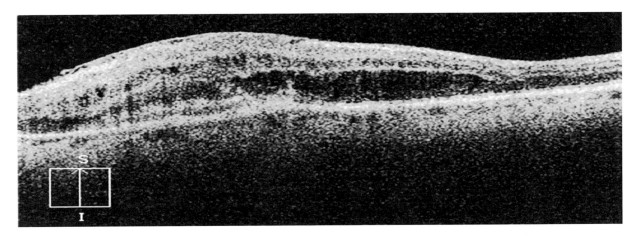

Epiretinal membrane outside the fovea causing traction retinal edema

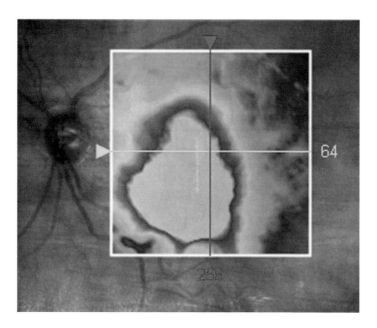

**An example of a volumetric OCT image from a patient with macular edema consistent with an epiretinal membrane**

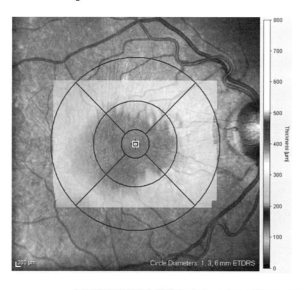

**Volumetric OCT of an ERM, both in false color designation and numeric values**

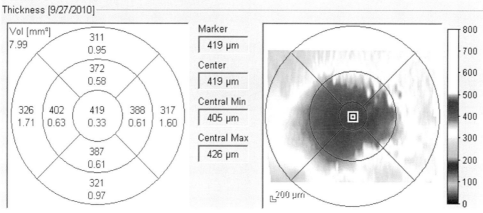

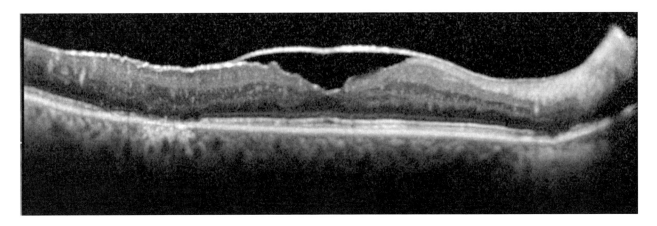

In this case, the epiretinal membrane spans the foveal depression, and is represented below on volumetric OCT as part of the retina. Therefore, it erroneously appears to the OCT software algorithm that there is a raised area of retina centrally

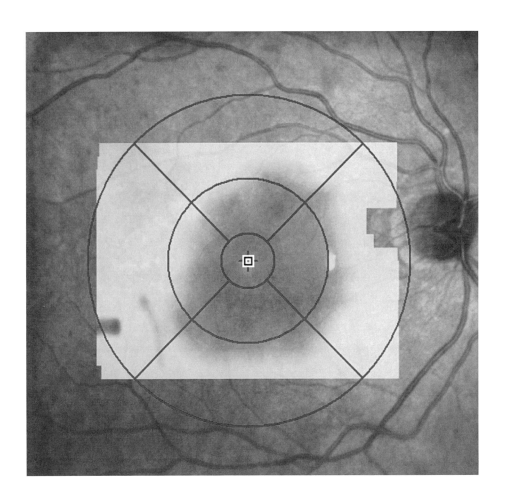

# Macular Holes

Because of the very nature of the pathology of a macular hole, patients may complain of a central visual defect. Relying on a patient's subjective fixation, they are asked to focus on a target that is preset in the OCT machine. This was discussed in the opening chapter, but should be mentioned again here. Patients with central vision defects will not be able to subjectively fixate with their anatomical fovea, and may fixate parafoveally, that is, outside of the fovea. The resulting scan will not image the fovea, but an area outside of the fovea. The imager must take into account the patient's visual history and complaint, and adjust the fixation target accordingly. More modern systems will track the patient's fovea, or even locate it for the imager, but that is not the case with all systems, and therefore the responsibility of scanning the proper area rests entirely on the imager. In the example on the following page, the first scan was done through the patient's subjective fixation. **(picture 1)** The imager then directs the patient to maintain fixation, and then moves the scan manually to find the area of interest; in this case, the fovea. **(picture 2)** The resulting images are drastically different, and may even alter the physician's diagnosis or the patient's treatment.

Don Gass originated the term macular hole in 1975. [14] With the advent of OCT and the ability to discern different retinal layers during the macular hole process, and differentiate full thickness macular holes, lamellar holes, pseudoholes and the retinal layers they affect allows scientists to re-evaluate original thinking. Typically lamellar holes have a thin fovea with avulsion of inner layers of the macula, [15] whereas full thickness macular holes open to the level of the RPE. With the help of OCT imaging, vitreomacular traction has been identified as one cause of full thickness and lamellar hole formation, [16] and in many cases of macular holes, epiretinal membranes are also present. [17] For the imager, macular holes present the very common problem of scanning the proper area of the retina, with limited and sometimes absent fixation assistance from the patient. This is another reason it is important for the imager to not accept the first subjective scan the system provides, but to move the scan to the appropriate location. Radial or raster scans that scan a large area of the macula are especially helpful to see the bigger picture, and to help narrow down the area of interest. The progression of macular holes is a unique disease entity that lends itself to sometimes spectacular OCT images.

Moving the scan outside the patient's subjective fixation often reveals different pathology:

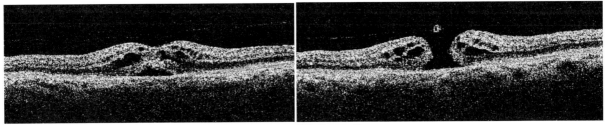

Picture 1                          Picture 2

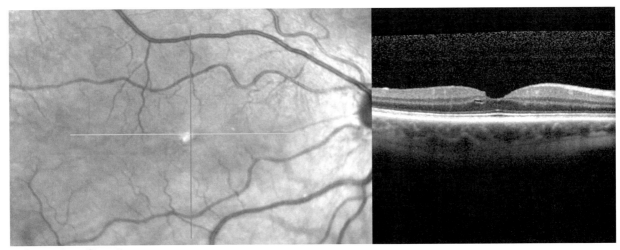

**Subjective fixation**

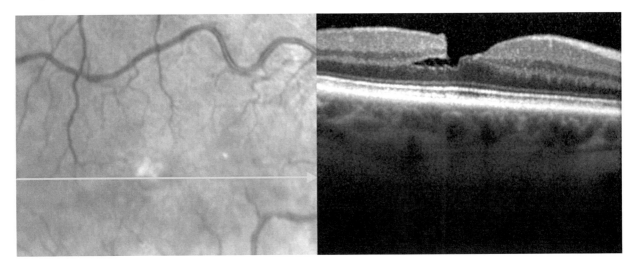

**After moving the scan**

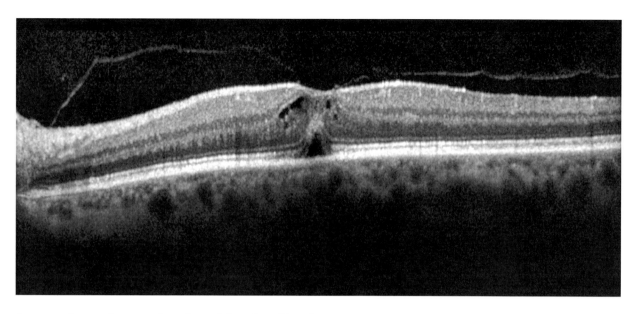

A scan through a patient's subjective fixation

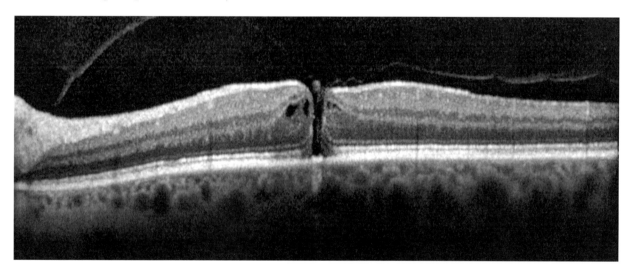

The same patient after the imager has moved the scan

Although the case above illustrates a very thin macular hole, it is a full thickness hole nonetheless. The first scan reveals a small "fluid" like space at the level of the RPE, which can be a clue to the imager that there is a full thickness hole present, and to move the scan.

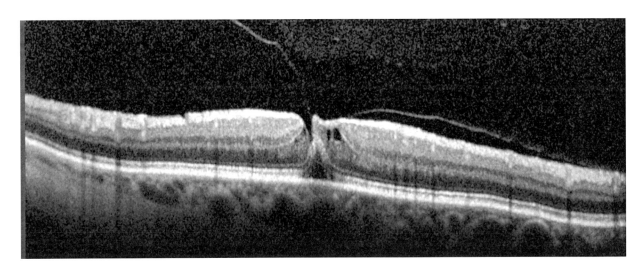

Another example of scanning through a patient's fixation. Note the telltale sign of vitreomacular traction

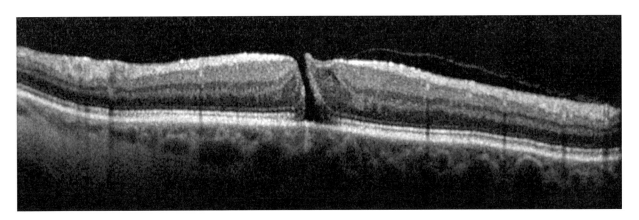

After moving the scan, a full thickness macular hole is revealed

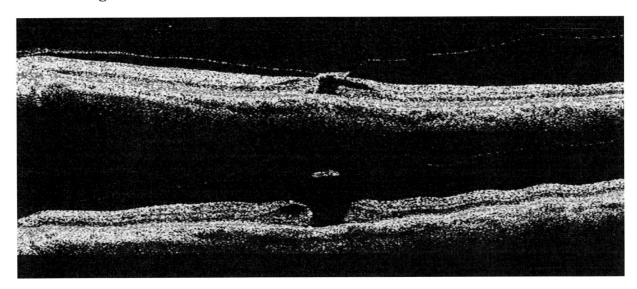

Macular traction (top) progressed to macular hole (bottom)

As was discussed previously in the segment on volumetric OCT, Time Domain OCT uses segmentary boundary lines to measure retinal volume or thickness. In the case of macular holes, this also presents a problem, as the boundary lines erroneously interpret the pattern as an area of elevation, not depression.

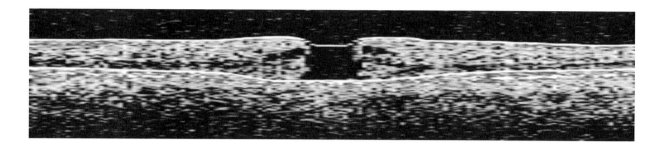

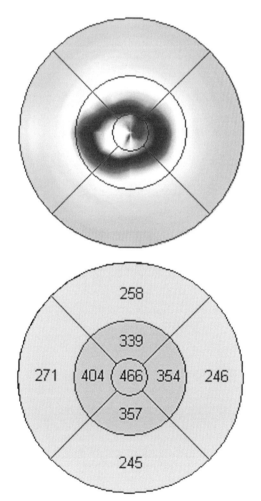

**Because of the segmentation line process of the volumetric analysis on Time Domain OCT, macular holes will be represented as an area of elevation, rather than excavation. Note the segmentation lines (in white) on the line scan that bridge across the macular hole**

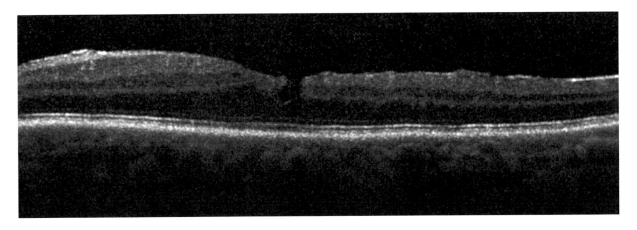

Partial thickness macular hole

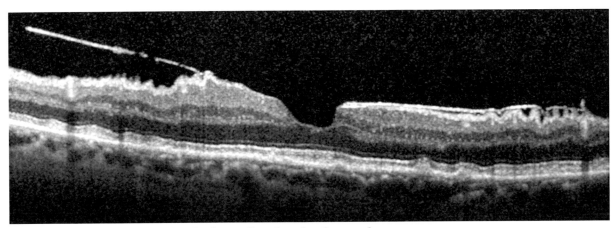

Partial thickness macular hole and epiretinal membrane

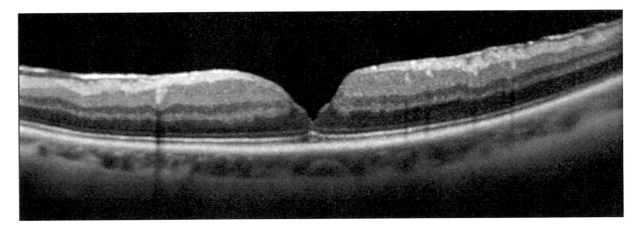

Partial thickness macular hole with minimal epiretinal membrane

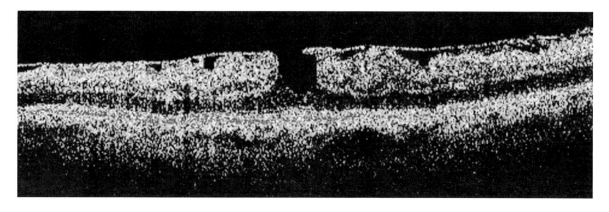

Lamellar hole with ERM on Time Domain OCT

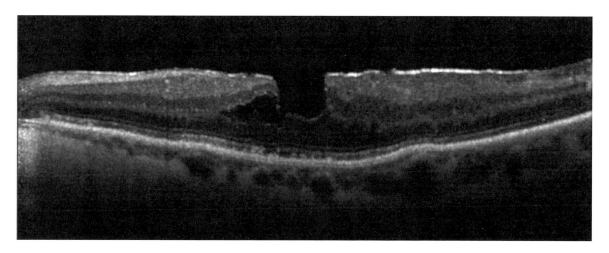

Partial thickness macular hole with hyper reflectivity of an ERM seen temporally

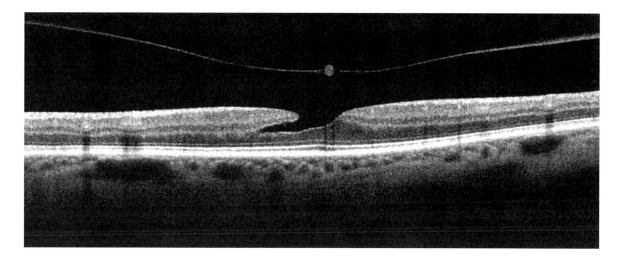

Partial thickness macular hole with operculum in vitreous interface

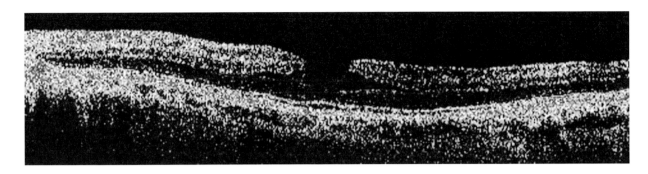

**Partial thickness macular hole on Time Domain OCT**

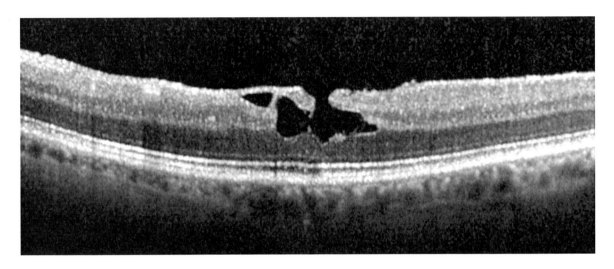

**Lamellar hole**

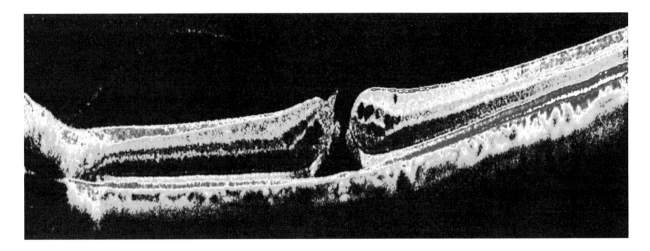

**Full thickness macular hole**

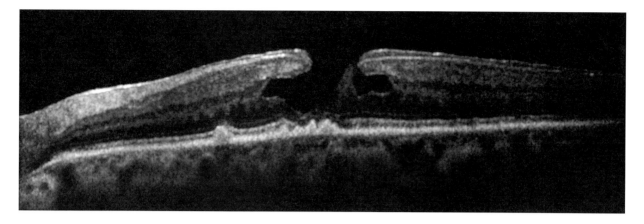

Pre op macular hole

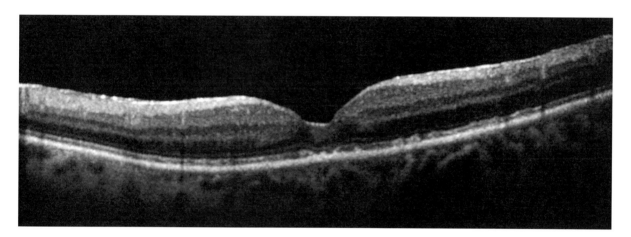

Post op macular hole

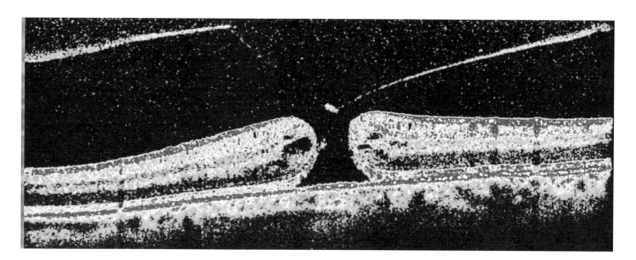

Full thickness macular hole with operculum

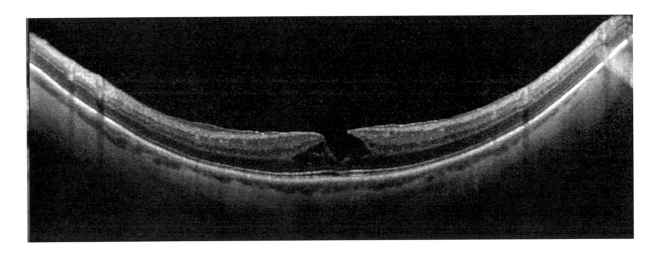

Partial thickness macular hole in high myope

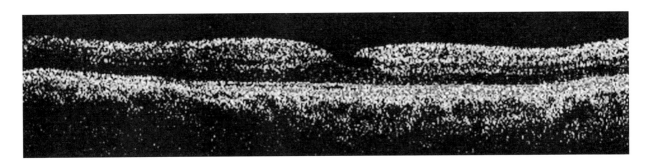

Partial thickness macular hole on Time Domain OCT

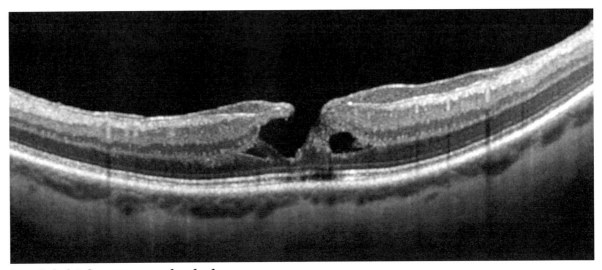

Partial thickness macular hole

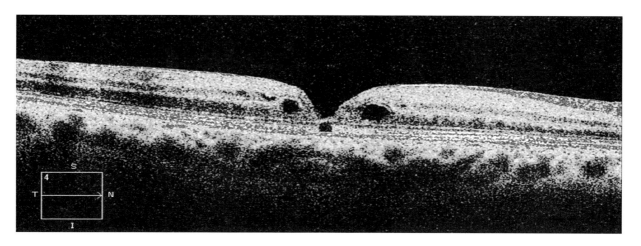

Partial thickness macular hole with associated edema

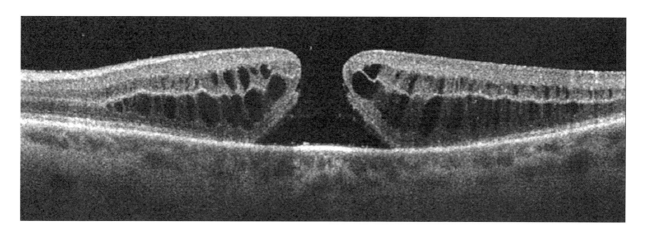

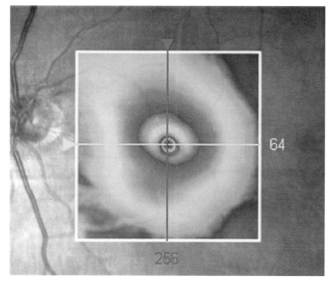

Volumetric display of macular hole on Spectral Domain. Note the excavation centrally, with elevated surrounding macula, represented by the red areas

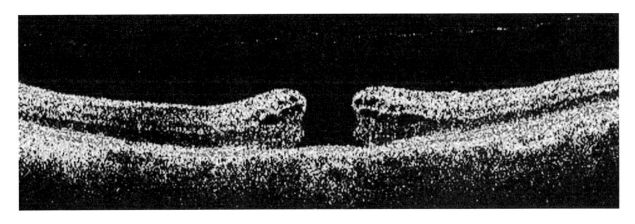

**Full thickness macular hole on Time Domain OCT**

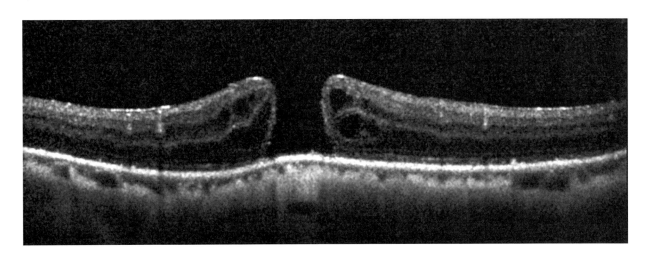

**Full thickness macular hole**

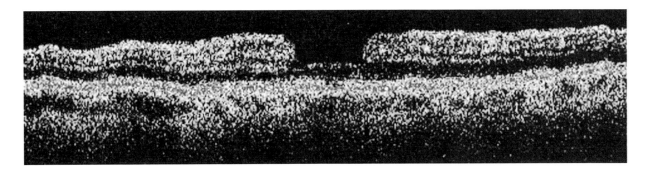

**Partial thickness macular hole on Time Domain OCT**

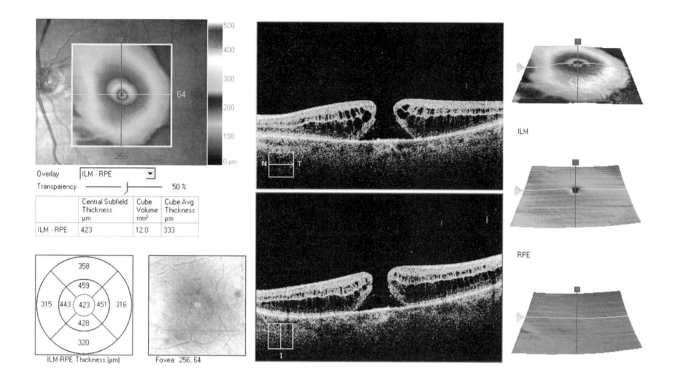

OCT display of full thickness macular hole with volumetric and individual layers presented

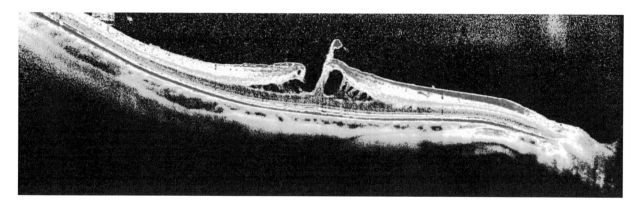

Partial thickness macular hole. Note residual tissue from vitreous traction

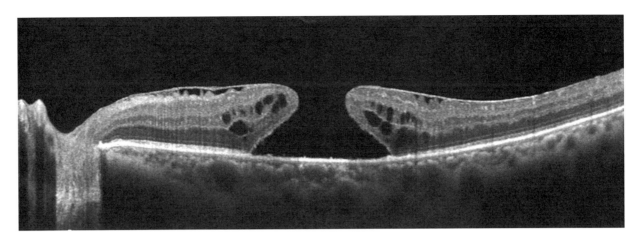

Full thickness macular hole with epiretinal membrane. Note the areas of intraretinal edema

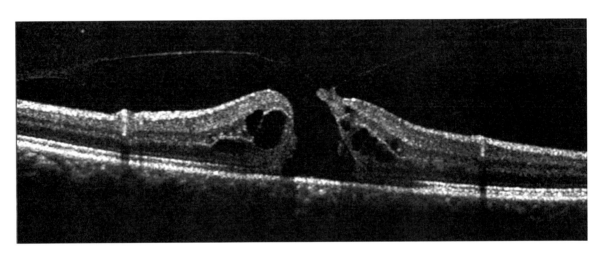

Full thickness macular hole with vitreomacular traction and macular edema

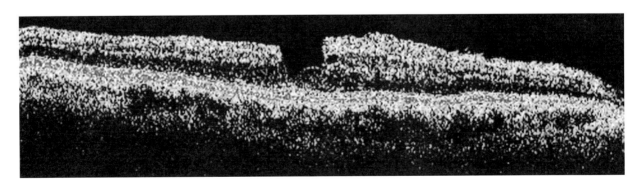

Partial thickness macular hole on Time Domain OCT

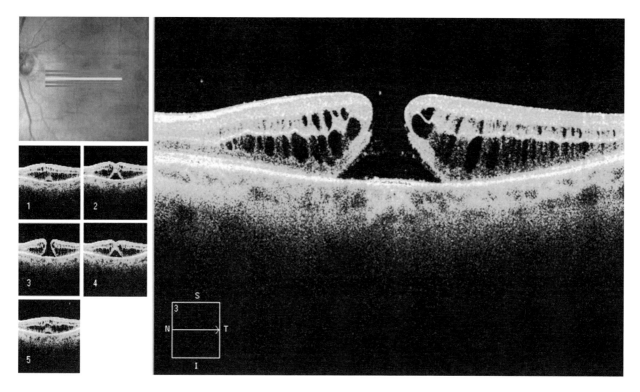

Full thickness macular hole. Top fundus image shows raster type scan, which uses multiple horizontal scans across a designated area

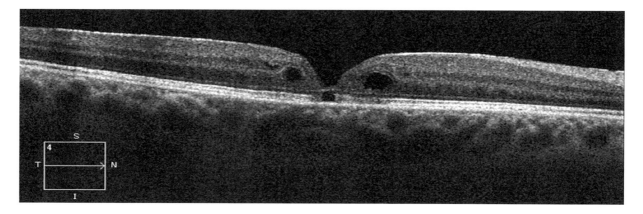

Lamellar hole with associated macular edema

A majority of OCT systems offer a preset crosshair or radial scan pattern that the imager can center on the fovea. In some instances, alternatively angled scans may better reveal pathology. In the example below, only presenting the horizontal scan does not offer the physician the entire story.

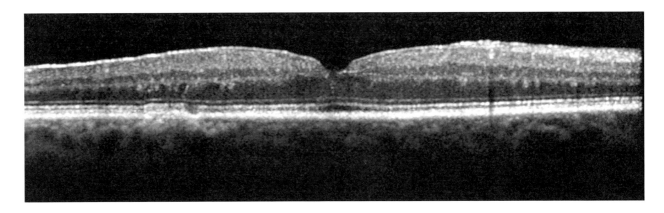

**Horizontal scan**

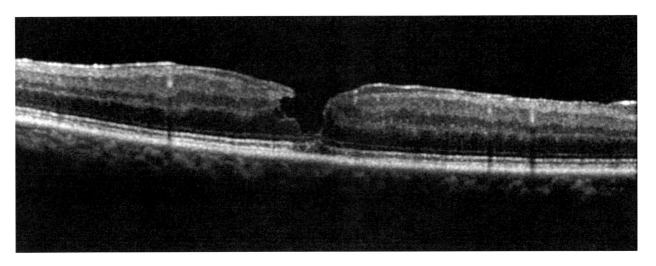

**Vertical scan, revealing a partial thickness macular hole with an epiretinal membrane**

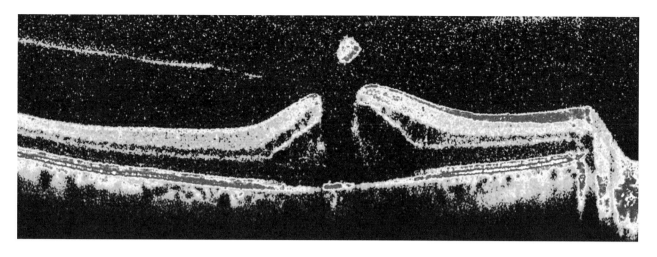

Full thickness macular hole with large operculum.  Note that the false color display in this image renders some separation of layers indistinguishable

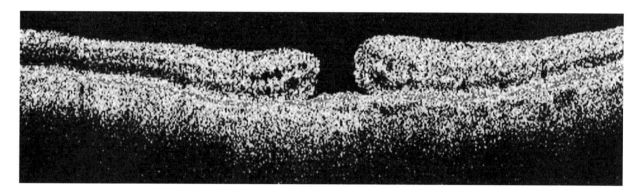

Full thickness macular hole on Time Domain OCT, with associated edema

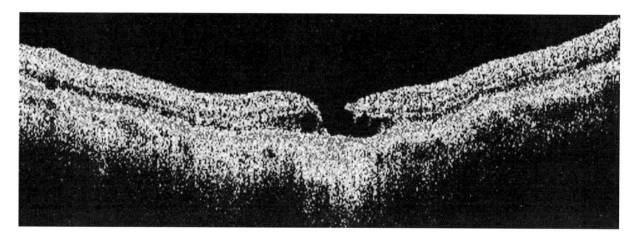

Full thickness macular hole on Time Domain OCT.  There is a highly reflective pattern under the fovea, indicating an area of atrophy or scar

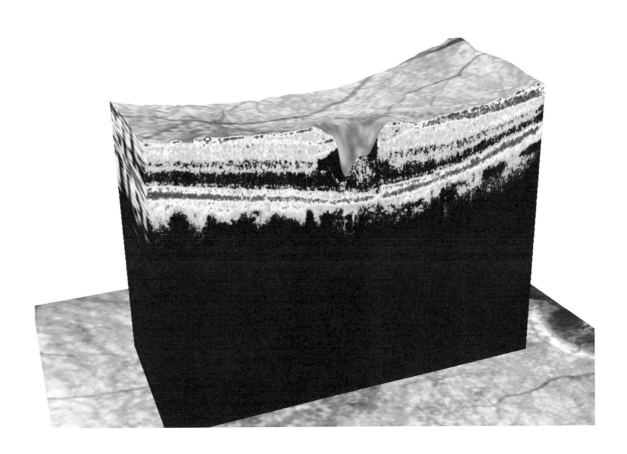

**3D cube OCT of a partial thickness macular hole**

# B. Intraretinal Pathology

As mentioned in the previous chapter, the intraretinal space is defined as above the interface of the photoreceptor layer and below the nerve fiber layer. Retinal disease that affects the intraretinal space typically presents as low-density reflectivity, and is usually attributed to fluid. Examples are diabetic macular edema, cystoid macular edema and edema resulting from retinal vein occlusion. Macular edema is defined as an abnormal thickening of the macula from excess fluid in the neurosensory retina. [18] The effects of vitreous traction and epiretinal membranes are seen in the intraretinal space as well, usually in the form of edema. These diseases rarely involve the sub retinal or sub-RPE space. Edema in the intraretinal space may be seen as singular oval or circular areas, or multiple petaloid type cystic spaces that respect clearly defined borders. Because the retinal blood vessels lie within the intraretinal tissue, breakdown or leakage of serous fluid or blood from these vessels are trapped within the layers of the intraretinal tissue. Separation of these tightly packed layers can cause disruption or distortion of the neural impulses being sent to the brain, resulting in visual disturbance. Frequently patients may complain of distortion of straight lines, general decrease in vision, and even loss of areas of vision.

Historically, before OCT, the only way to image macular edema, aside from ophthalmoscopy, was fluorescein angiography. Angiography would reveal either a late petaloid leakage pattern or a diffuse leakage of dye in the intraretinal layer (see image on next page). Evaluation of treatment or serial angiograms was done to subjectively estimate the decrease or increase of dye in the intraretinal space. With OCT, both line and volumetric scans of macular edema can be used to quantify the volume of fluid in the intraretinal space. With most systems, the software can show difference in the volume of edema between scans.

In Spectral Domain OCT and occasionally Time Domain OCT, retinal vessels, which lie in the intraretinal layer, can be clearly defined. Because of their reflectivity and density, these vessels will cast a shadow posteriorly, sometimes obscuring detail as far down as the choroid. This is true of any dense pathology, such as intraretinal hemorrhages or vitreous debris.

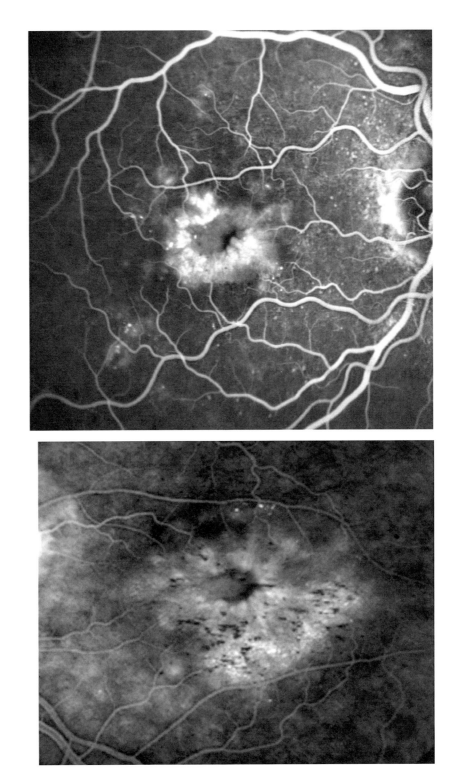

Fluorescein angiogram images of CME. Note the petaloid, cystic type spaces around the fovea that are hyperfluorescent from leakage of fluorescein dye

## Cystoid Macular Edema (CME)

Cystoid macular edema is an accumulation of intraretinal fluid in the macula with the formation of cystic spaces. Usually, the edema is a result of breakdown of the inner blood-retinal barrier and leakage of plasma from capillaries. [19] In some cases, it can be associated with post cataract surgery, and is labeled as Irvine-Gass syndrome. [20] OCT is particularly useful for imaging this disease, as it can clearly outline the cystic spaces in the intraretinal tissue, and can, in many cases, replace fluorescein angiography as the clinical standard for imaging CME. OCT can also be used to track or follow the course of treatment, not only for CME, but for other pathology. The systems available allow serial scans to be taken over a period of time, and the software can compare and display volumetric change values in a quantitative fashion.

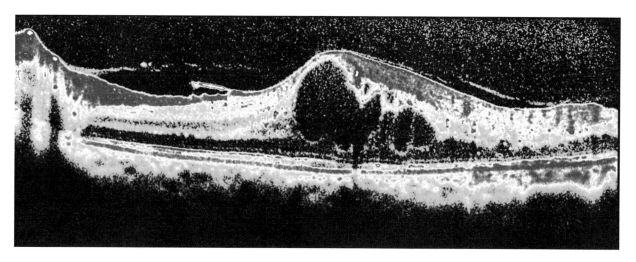

**Typical cystoid macular edema with oblong, cystic spaces in the fovea**

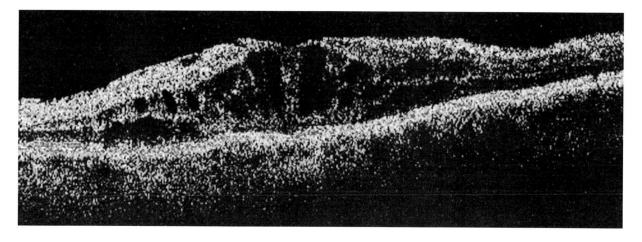

**CME on Time Domain OCT**

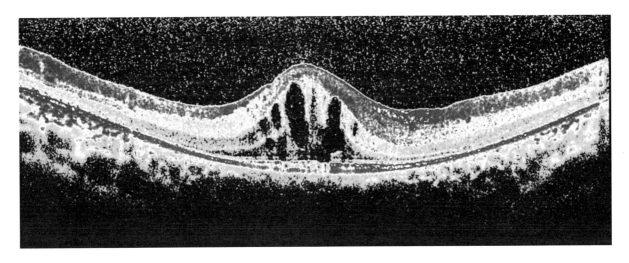

Spectral domain OCT of CME

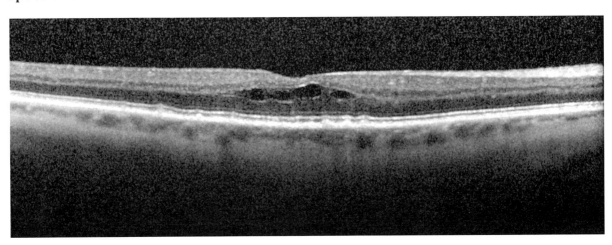

CME can sometimes obscure the foveal depression

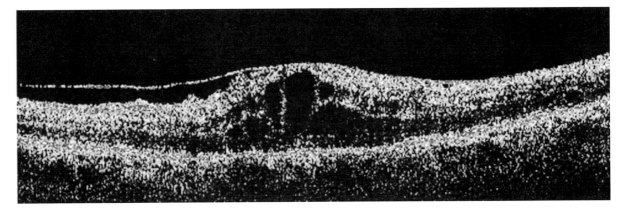

CME with an epiretinal membrane, possibly causing traction, which compounds the pathology

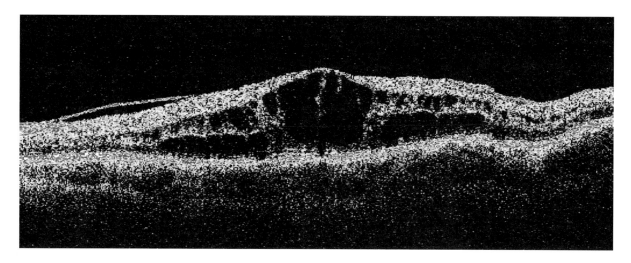

CME with epiretinal membrane on Time Domain OCT

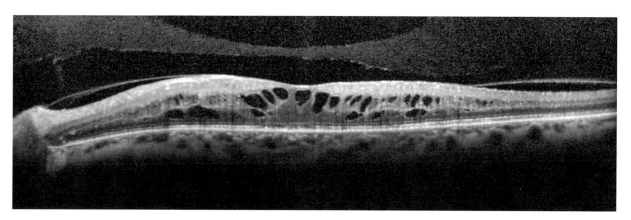

Multiple cystic spaces as well as a partial posterior vitreous detachment

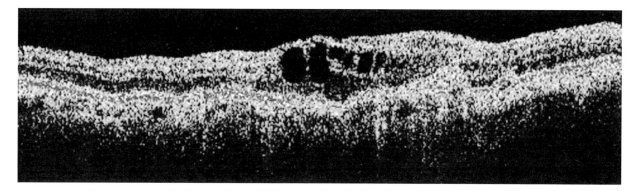

Time Domain OCT

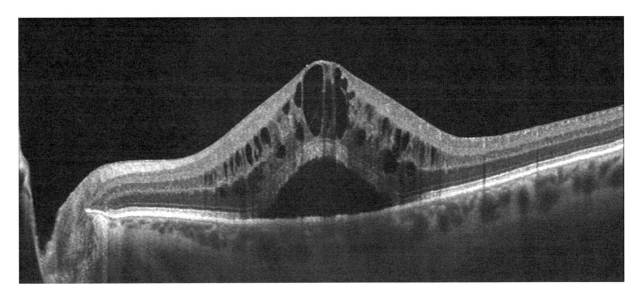

Severe CME with associated sub retinal fluid

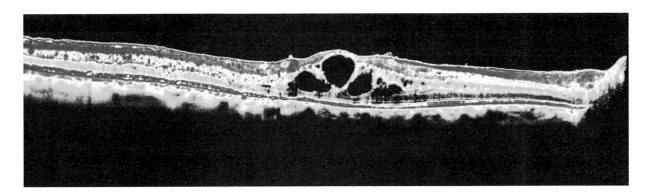

Colored Spectral Domain OCT of CME with typical cystic, petaloid pattern spaces

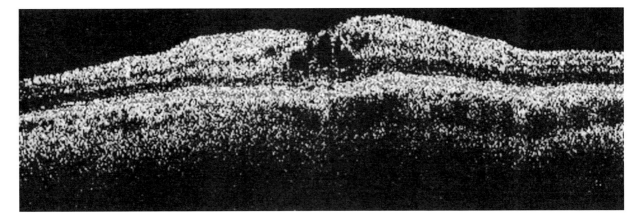

CME in a typical petaloid pattern on Time Domain OCT

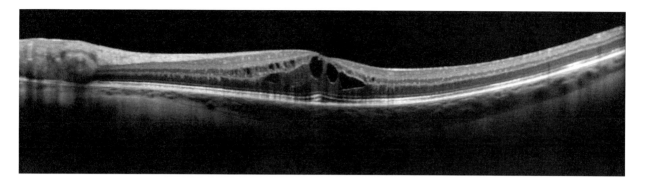

CME, demonstrated in several layers of intraretinal tissue

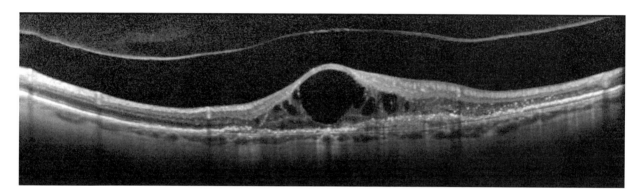

Large macular cyst with CME and posterior vitreous detachment

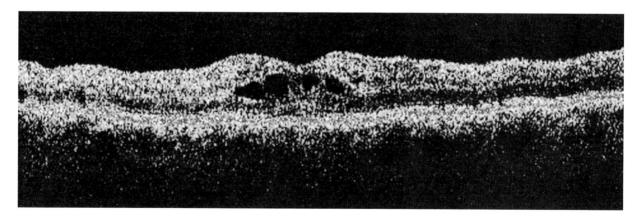

CME on Time Domain OCT

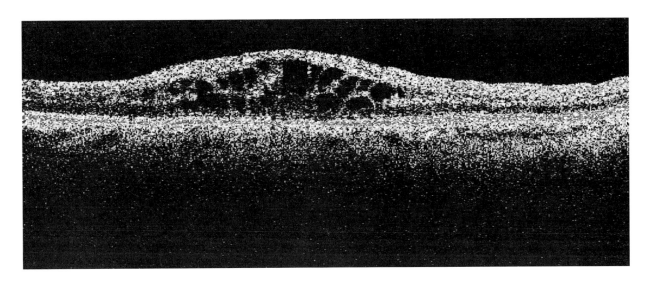

CME demonstrated on Time Domain OCT

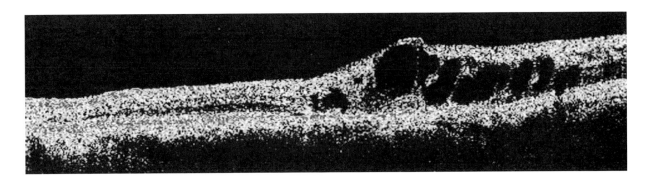

CME image on Time Domain OCT

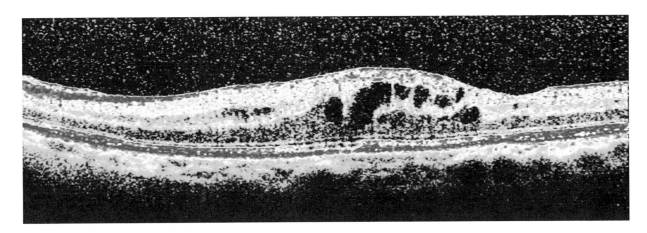

CME may distort the macula and make it difficult to locate a foveal depression

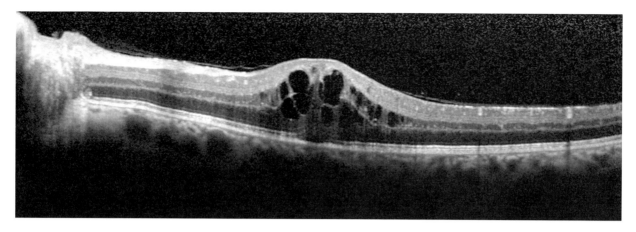

CME with lipid exudates

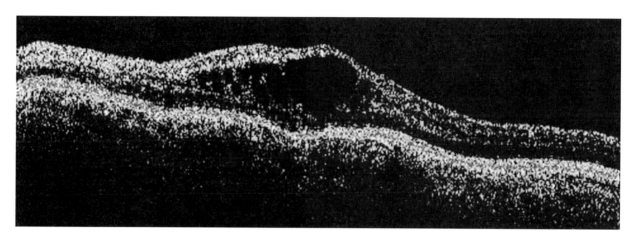

In some cases, the fovea may be so elevated that multiple scans must be taken to best represent the pathology

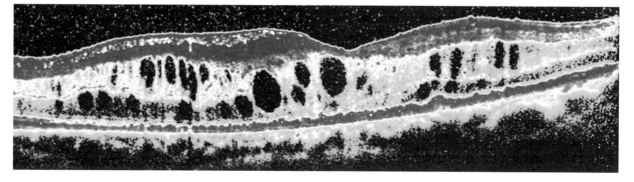

Chronic CME

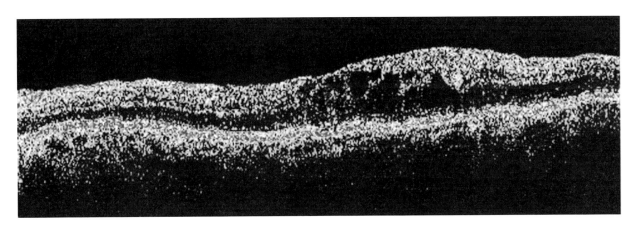

Cystoid macular edema on Time Domain OCT, with corresponding volumetric OCT below. Note the area of fluid is mostly temporal, as reflected on the volumetric analysis

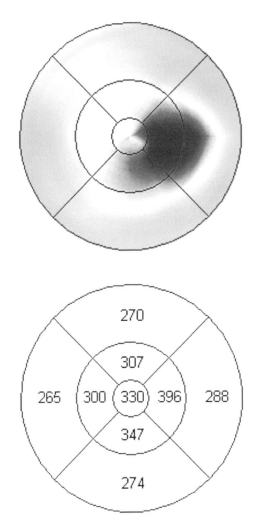

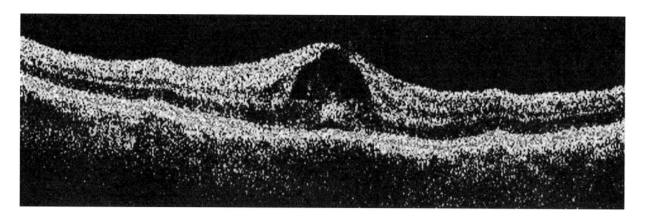

Large macular cyst on Time Domain OCT

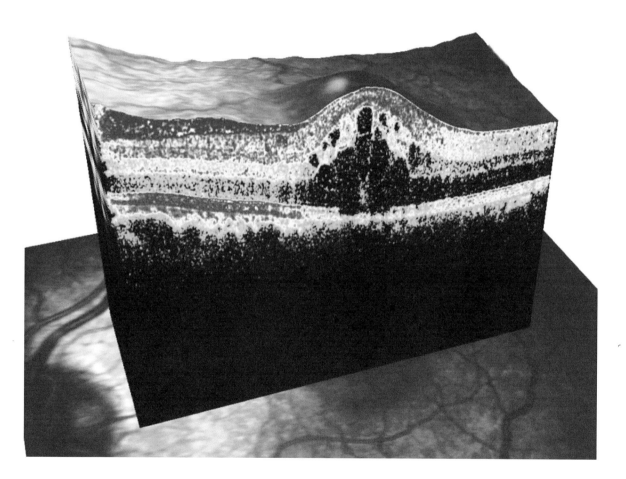

Three-dimensional cube showing CME and elevated macula

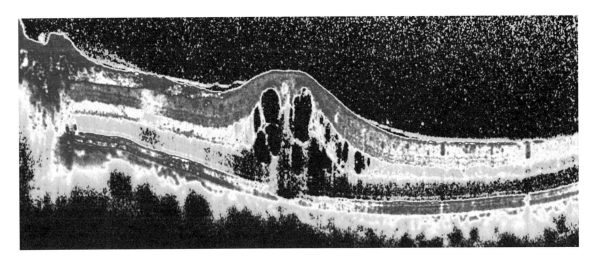

**Diffuse CME**

## Diabetic Macular Edema (DME)

Another common form of macular edema results from diabetic retinopathy. This type of edema may present at any level of diabetic retinopathy, and occurs in about 10% of patients with diabetes. 21 DME may present like CME, with cystic spaces of fluid within the intraretinal space, but there may also be hard exudates present. Because of their density, they are represented on OCT as brighter reflective pathology. 22 These exudates are derived from leaking microaneurysms, and are found mostly in the outer and inner plexiform layers. Diabetic macular edema is mostly due to leaking microaneurysms, a condition regularly found in patients with diabetic retinopathy. The leakage occurs within the tightly packed layers of the intraretinal space and causes separation of these layers. 23

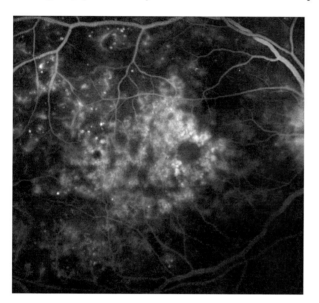 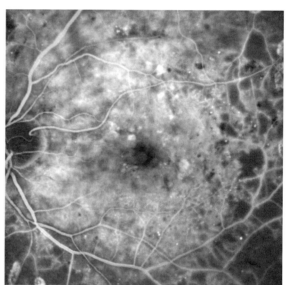

**Fluorescein angiogram of two diabetic patients with diabetic macular edema. Note the areas of hyperfluorescence that are represented on OCT as pockets of fluid within the intraretinal space**

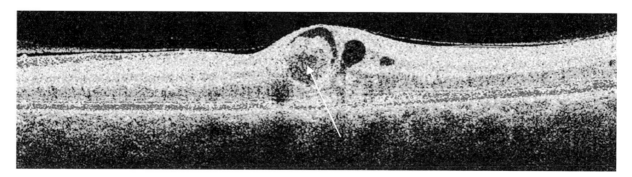

**DME with large lipid exudates (white arrow)**

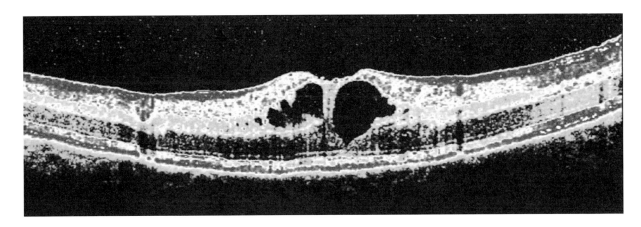

Diabetic macular edema presented as cystic spaces around the fovea

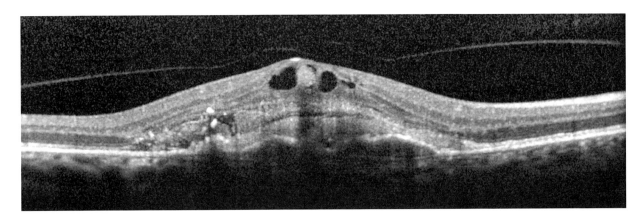

DME with highly elevated macula

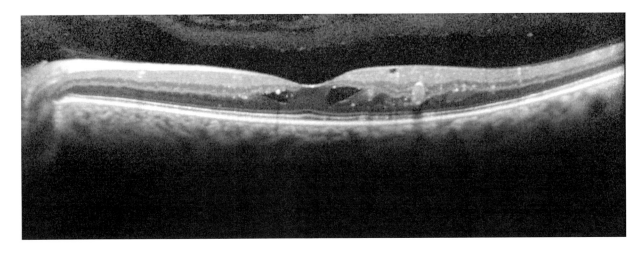

DME with posterior vitreous detachment (unrelated)

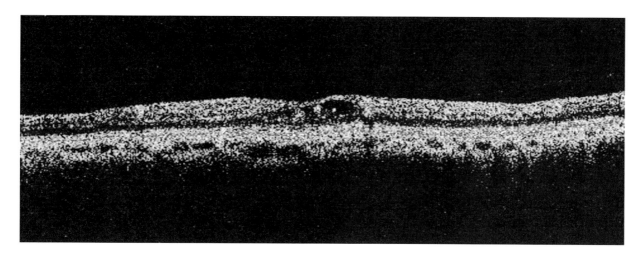

DME on Time domain OCT, which can be difficult to image fluid spaces

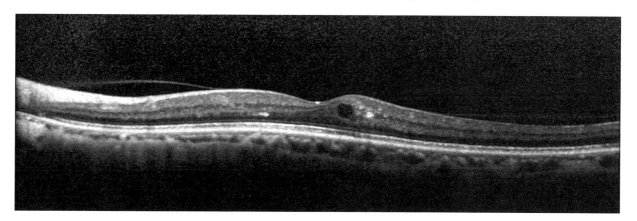

Spectral domain OCT image of the same patient as above

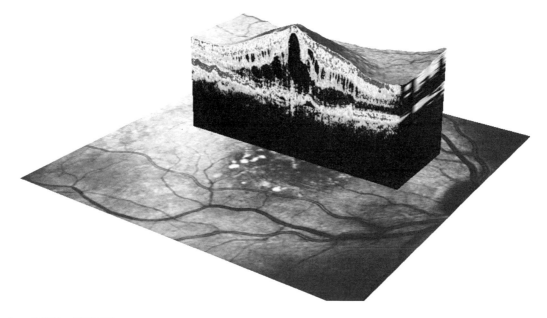

3D cube OCT of DME

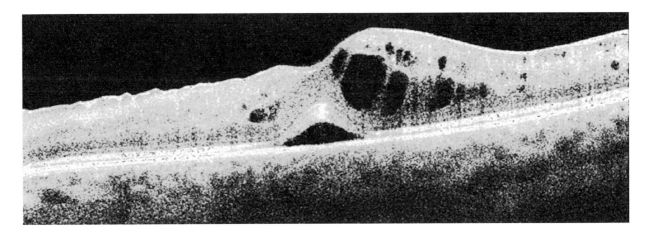

DME with sub retinal fluid

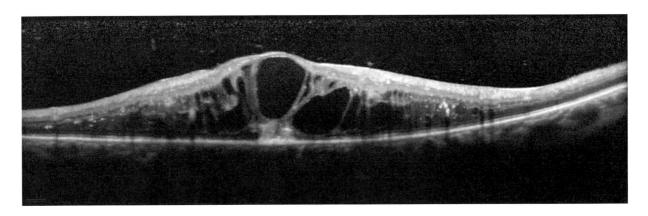

Multiple areas of cystic spaces within the intraretinal space

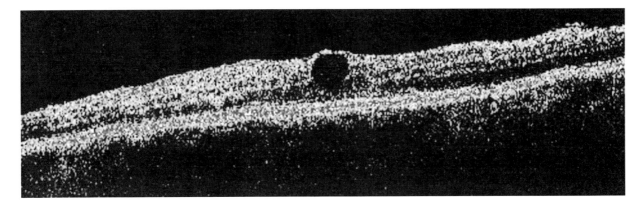

Large macular cyst

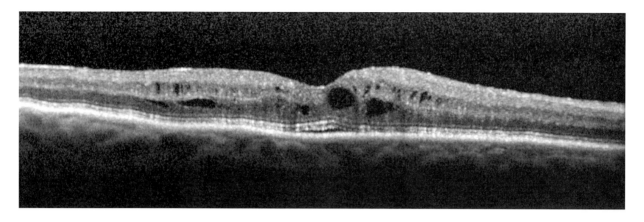

Multiple areas of cystic spaces, both in the fovea and extrafoveally

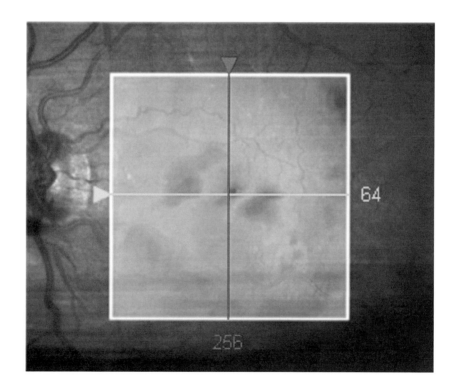

Volumetric OCT of DME. Note the areas of edema, marked by red in this image

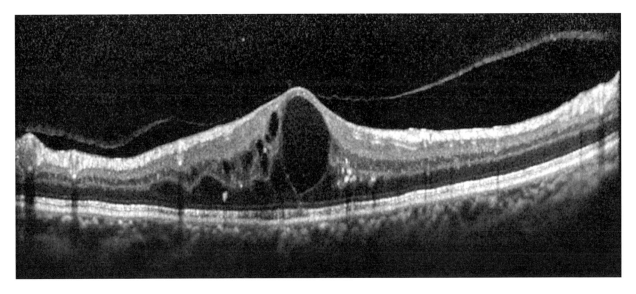

DME with large macular cyst. There is vitreous traction as well, but because the vitreous interface is not taut, the edema is attributed to diabetic retinopathy

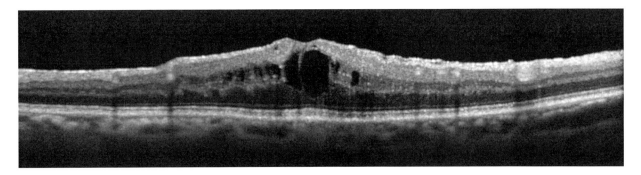

**Cystic pockets under the fovea**

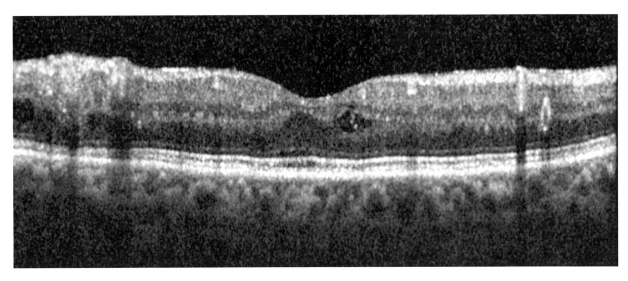

**DME and hard exudates**

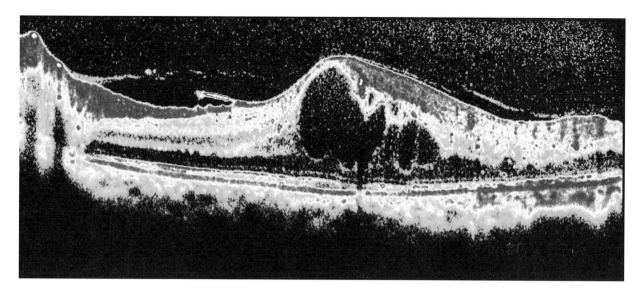

**Multiple cystic pockets of fluid**

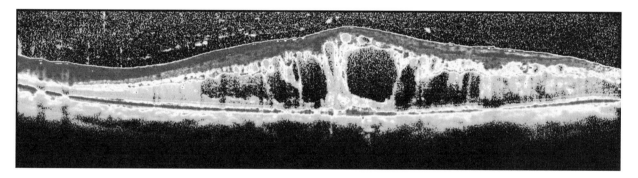

**Large area of edema in the macula**

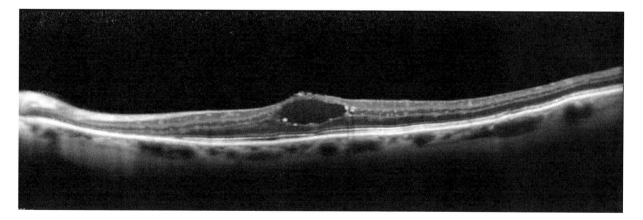

**Large macular cyst**

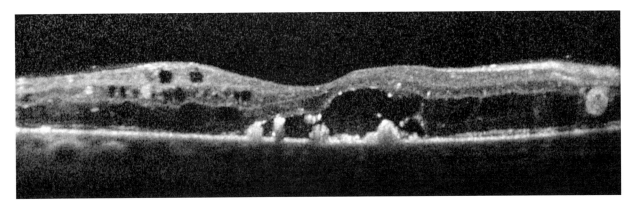

DME with hard drusen, represented by the hyper reflective areas just above the RPE

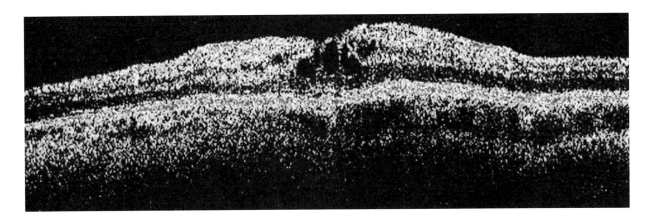

DME on Time Domain OCT

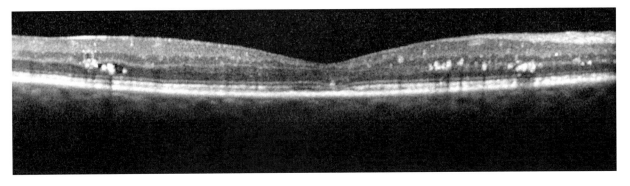

Diabetic with resolved macular edema, but residual lipid exudates-represented by the hyper reflective material within the intraretinal space

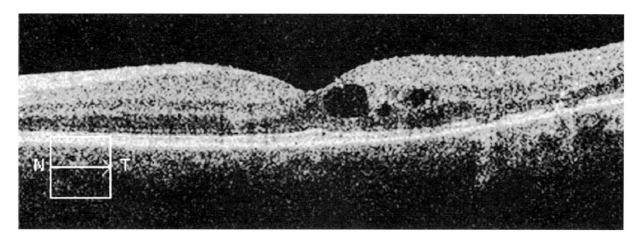

Large cystic space just temporal to the fovea and multiple smaller spaces of fluid

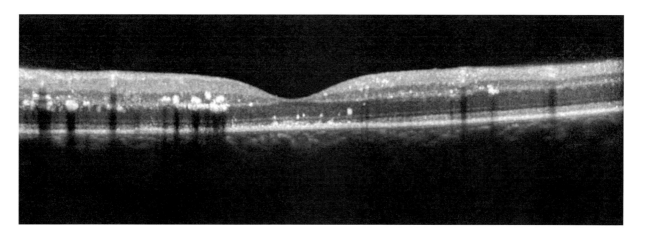

DME with lipid exudates. Note the hyper reflectivity of the exudates

**DME on Time Domain with corresponding volumetric OCT analysis**

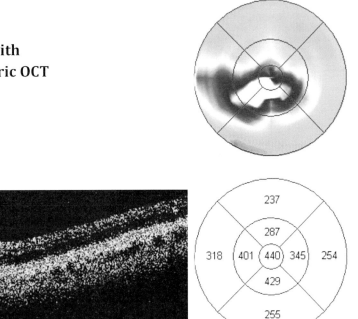

Vertical Time Domain scan, demonstrating fluid inferior to the fovea, as also seen on volumetric OCT

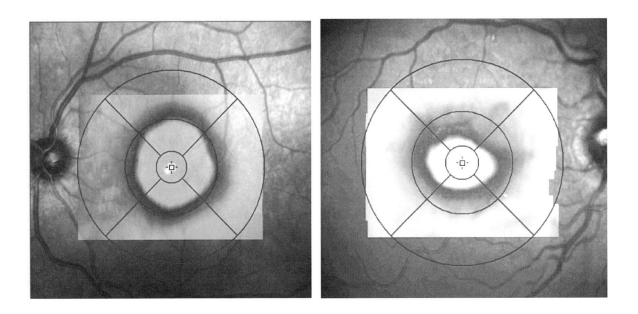

**Volumetric OCT of two patients with DME**

# Retinal Vein Occlusions

Retinal vein occlusion (RVO) is the most common retinal vascular disease after diabetic retinopathy [24] and macular edema is a frequent cause of vision loss in eyes with RVO. [25] RVO is likely caused by a thrombotic event. In the case of Central Retinal Vein Occlusion, this may occur in the central vein at the lamina cribrosa. In Branch Retinal Vein Occlusion, this happens at an arteriovenous crossing, that is, where an artery crosses a vein. The artery may compress the vein and increase turbulent flow, which in turn increases intraluminal pressure and transudation of blood products into the retina, causing increased retinal fluid. [26] Hypertension is the strongest risk factor for developing retinal vein occlusion. [27] OCT is a great clinical tool for not only imaging the extent of macular edema caused by RVO, but to quantify change over time or after treatment. Fluorescein angiography is typically used in tandem with OCT, not necessarily to evaluate edema, but to also evaluate ischemia from RVO and to evaluate reperfusion of the vein(s).

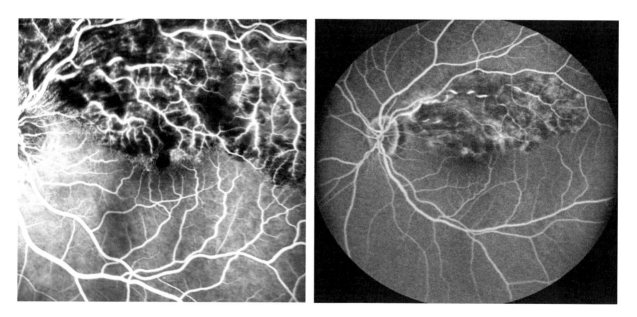

**Two cases of branch retinal vein occlusion on fluorescein angiography**

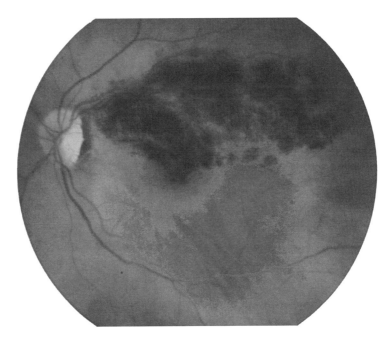

Color fundus photograph of a branch retinal vein occlusion

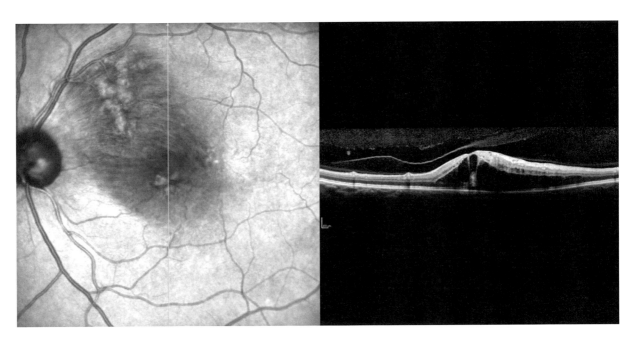

Vertical OCT scan through the fovea with the area of vein occlusion and edema superiorly

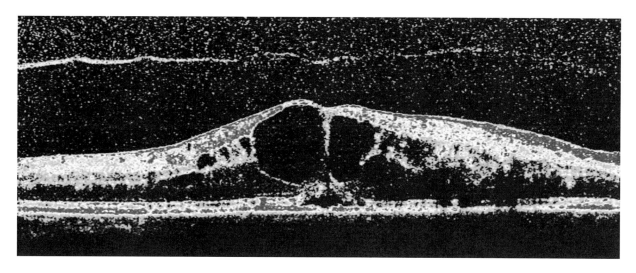

Macular edema due to RVO

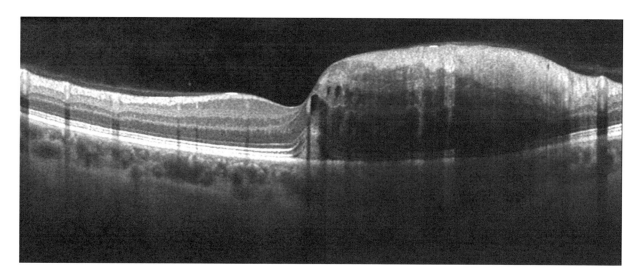

Vertical OCT scan showing edema in the superior macula

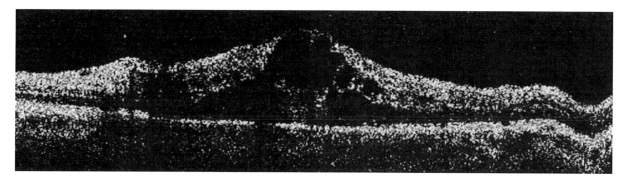

Time domain OCT of macular edema from retinal vein occlusion

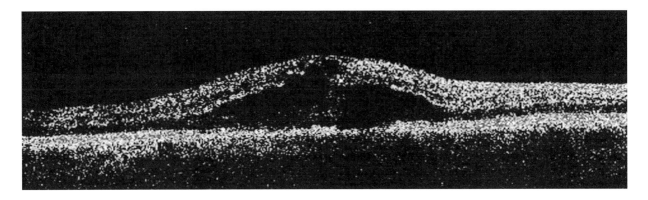

RVO on Time domain OCT

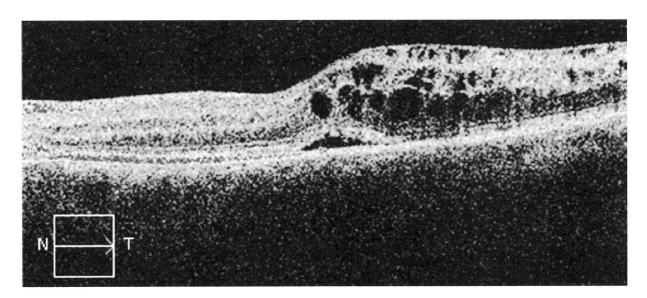

Spectral domain OCT image of temporal macular edema from RVO

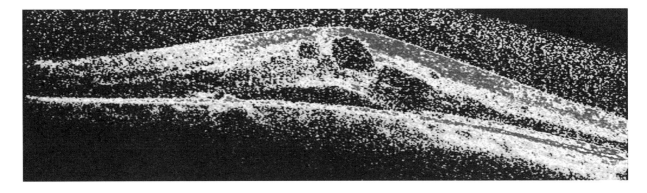

RVO with intraretinal edema and sub retinal fluid

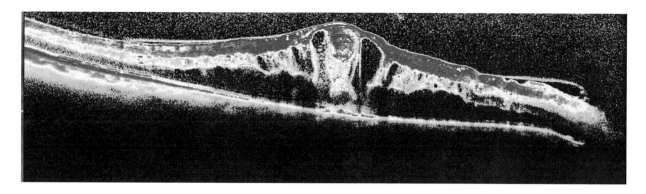

**Severe edema throughout the macula from RVO**

Although edema from RVO can affect the central macula and fovea, in the following examples the OCT image reflects edema on one side of the macula.

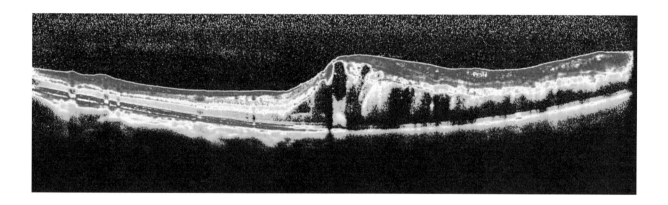

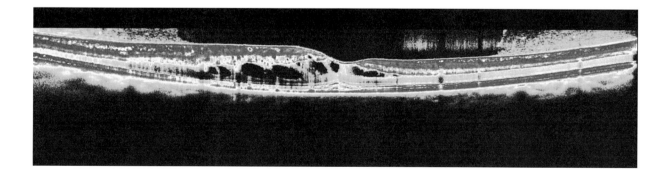

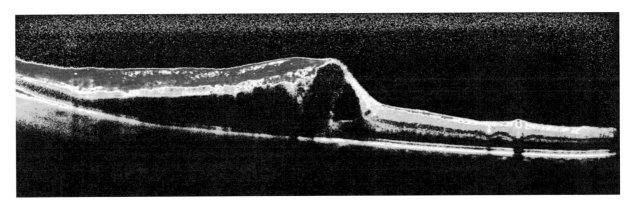

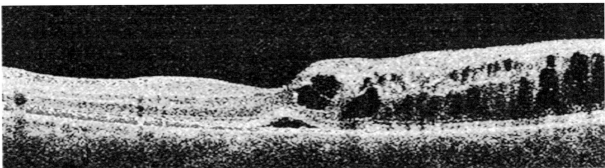

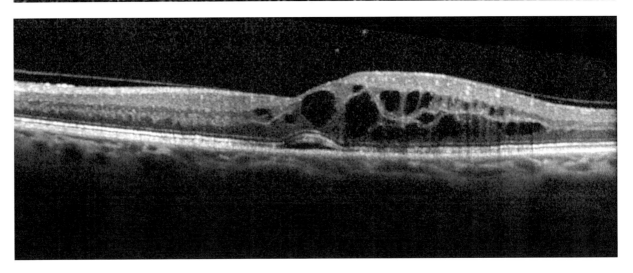

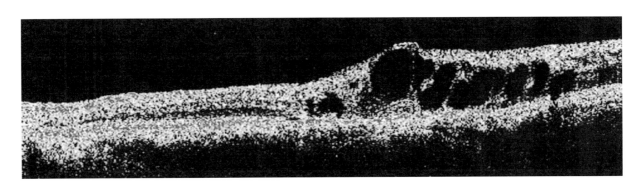

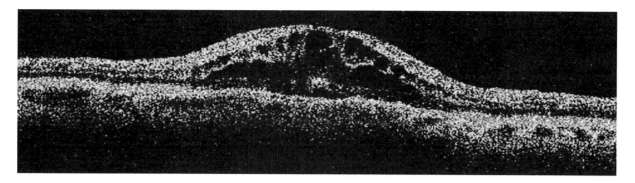

Large central area of macula edema due to vein occlusion

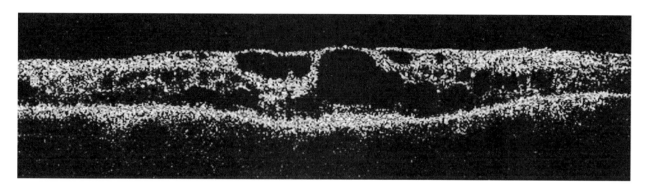

Vein occlusion with epiretinal membrane

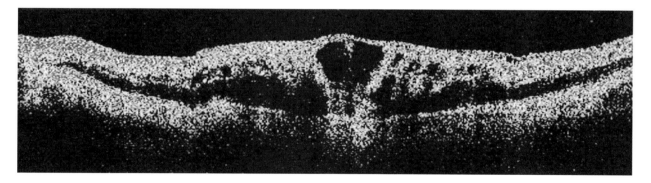

Multiple areas of edema, with large cysts in fovea

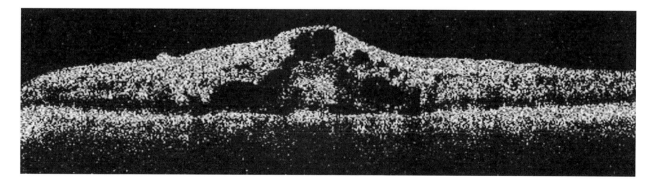

Time Domain OCT of multiple areas of edema

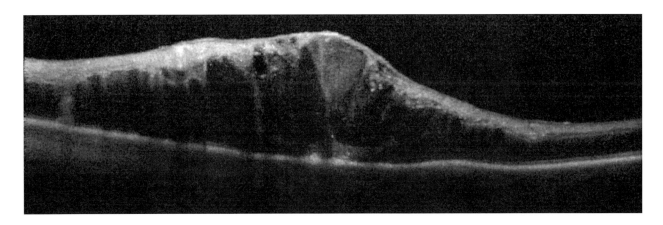

Substantial edema due to vein occlusion

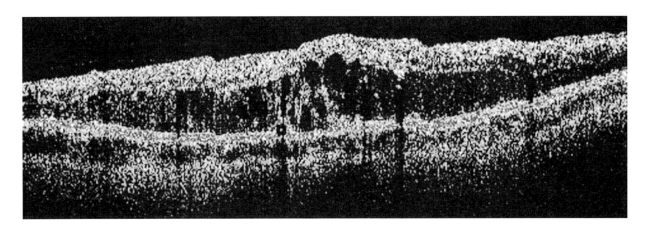

Large area of edema from vein occlusion, with multiple hyper reflective areas of lipid

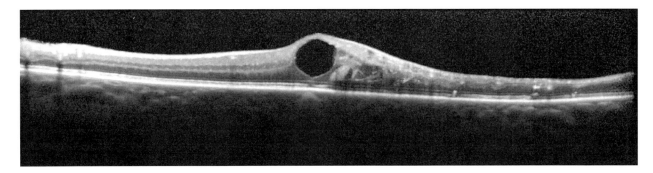

Single large cyst of edema in the fovea, with smaller areas of edema temporally

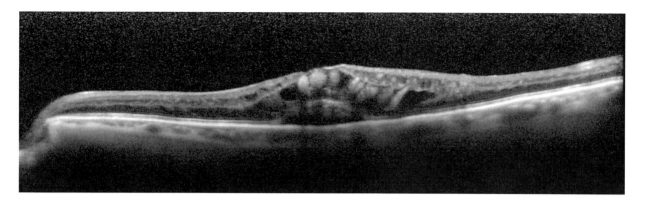

RVO with multiple areas of cystic edema

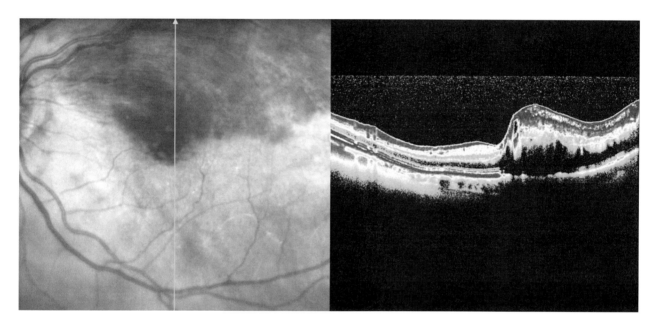

Vertical OCT scan with corresponding fundus image showing superior vein occlusion

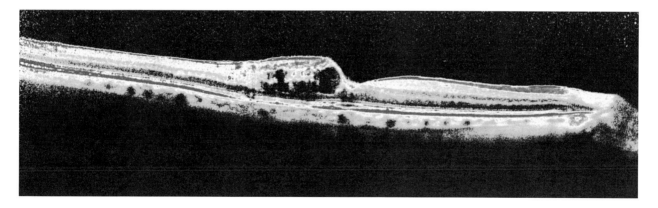

Horizontal OCT scan with edema temporally

## C. Sub RPE and Sub Retinal Pathology

Retinal disease that affect the sub RPE and sub retina, such as macular degeneration and central serous retinopathy, typically presents as low density reflectivity (such as fluid) and high density reflectivity (such as CNV, scar or drusen).

## Macular Degeneration

Macular degeneration is the leading cause of blindness in Americans 55 and older, affecting more than 10 million. [28] Classified as either "wet" or "dry" macular degeneration, it is one of the most imaged retinal diseases in practices. OCT allows the operator to image the very fine layers that AMD affects, mainly the RPE, Bruch's membrane and the choriocapillaris. Dry AMD is defined as a progressive thinning of the RPE and area tissue, which may lead to geographic atrophy. Patients may complain of decreased vision and metamorphopsia, and at this time, there is no treatment for dry AMD. [29] The wet form of AMD occurs when new blood vessels, usually from the choroid, spread through breaks in Bruch's membrane and infiltrate the sub RPE and sub retinal space. Choroidal vessels are naturally fenestrated, so blood products leak into the retinal tissue, and cause localized detachments of the layers of retina. A patient with this form of AMD typically presents with a rapid decrease in vision, and areas of vision that may be missing. There are a multitude of treatments for wet AMD at this time, and more treatments are being studied.

Early stages of AMD may include drusen, which may be an indicator of increased risk of progression to advanced AMD. [30] OCT is an excellent clinical tool for the baseline evaluation of AMD, as well as on-going serial imaging for the treatment of choroidal neovascularization in AMD. As modern treatment of choroidal neovascularization typically requires monthly evaluation to determine the need for retreatment, [31] OCT may replace fluorescein angiography for the follow up of exudative AMD. [32]

## Drusen

Drusen are typically small deposits under the RPE but above Bruch's Membrane and can be classified as soft or hard. Soft drusen are described as deposits that have indistinct borders and tend to be larger, and may be a precursor to macular degeneration, whereas hard drusen have distinct borders and tend to be smaller than 63 microns. [33]

On OCT, drusen appear distinctly under the RPE and, as with all pathology, hyper reflectivity depends on the density of the drusen. Soft drusen appear less reflective, or greyer, and hard drusen are more reflective, and appear whiter.

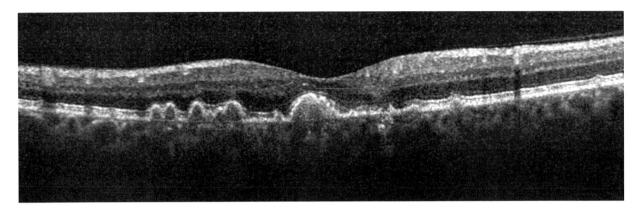

**In this case, there are multiple drusen throughout the macula, with a large druse under the fovea**

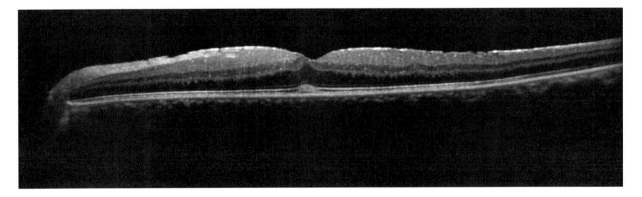

**Note the hyper reflectivity of the druse under the fovea. This is indicative of a denser or hard druse**

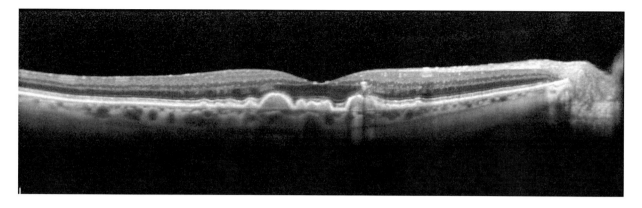

Less hyper reflectivity under the RPE indicates soft drusen

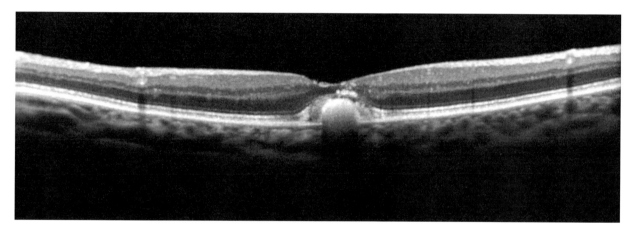

Drusen may be so dense that the OCT laser signal may be obscured after passing through the pathology

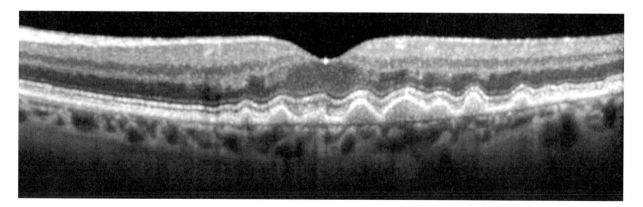

Multiple large soft drusen

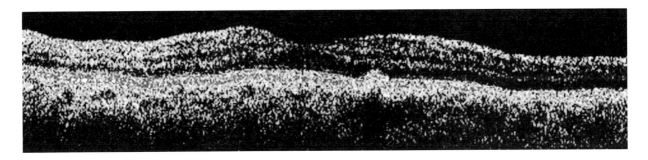

**Time Domain OCT of a single druse**

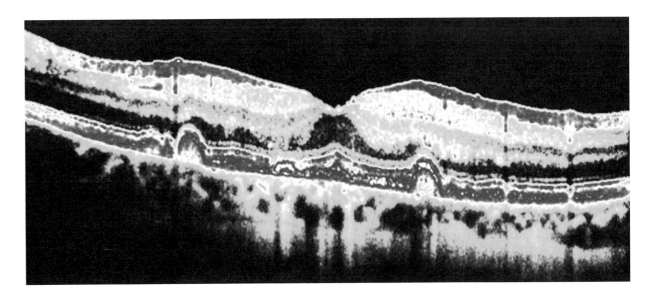

**Multiple soft drusen**

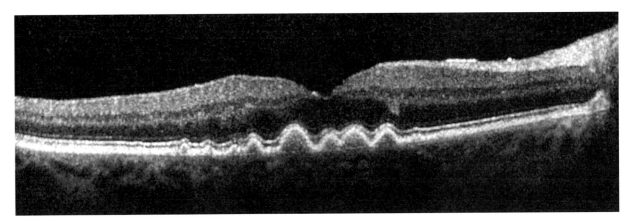

**Multiple soft drusen**

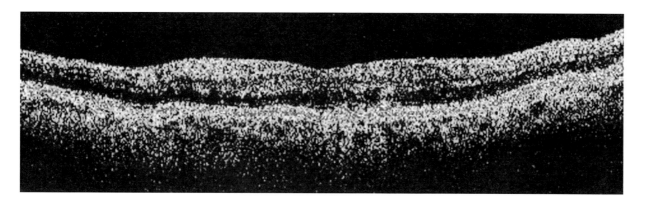

Time Domain OCT of multiple drusen under the fovea

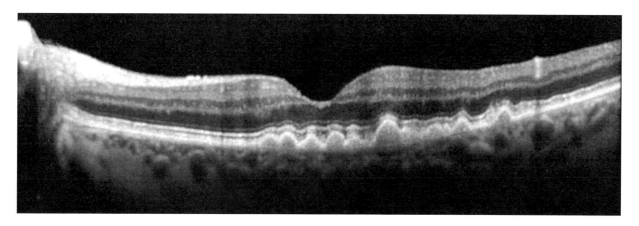

Multiple soft drusen

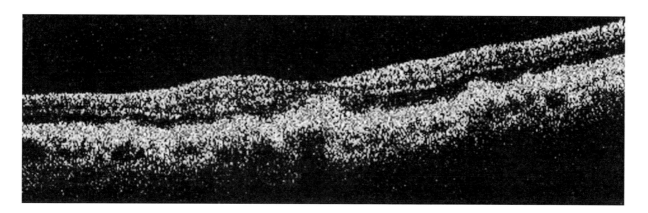

Multiple drusen with a large druse under the fovea on Time Domain OCT

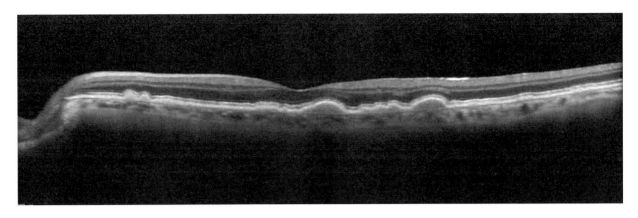

Several large soft drusen and a few small soft drusen

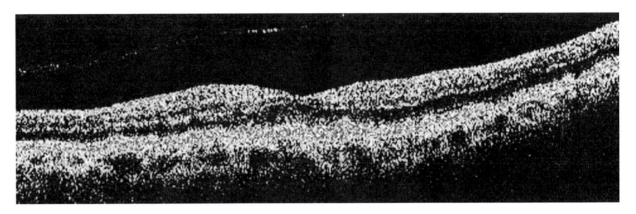

Multiple small drusen throughout the macula

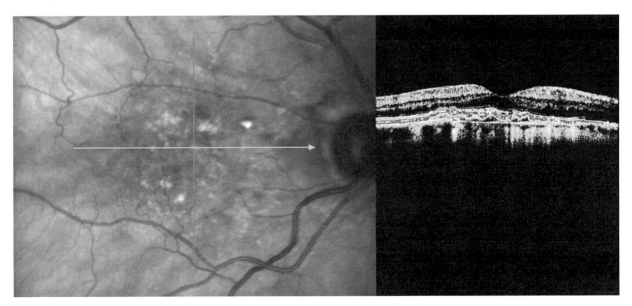

Multiple soft drusen on fundus image and corresponding OCT image

## Reticular Pseudodrusen

Described in many publications, reticular pseudodrusen are best imaged either with the blue channel of color fundus photography or with infrared wavelength, as seen in the images below. On OCT, the pseudodrusen appear as hyper reflective material <u>above</u> the RPE, in the sub retinal space between the RPE and the boundary between inner and outer segments of the photoreceptors. [34]

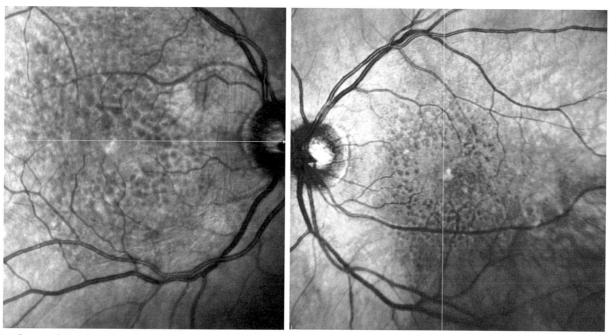

**Infrared and color image of pseudodrusen. Note the speckled pattern of drusen throughout the macula**

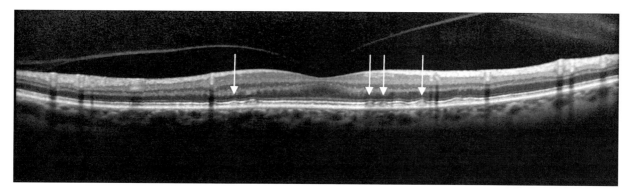

**Reticular pseudodrusen appear between the RPE and the boundary between inner and outer segments of the photoreceptors (arrows)**

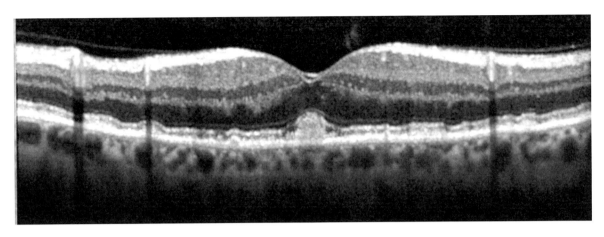

Reticular pseudodrusen and a large druse under the fovea

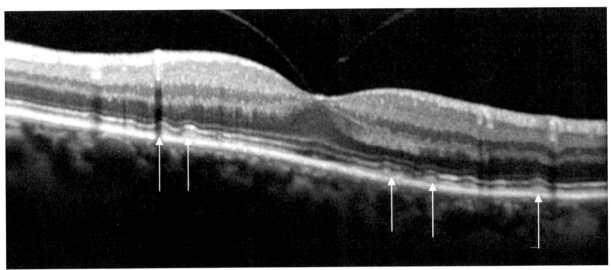

Reticular pseudodrusen and vitreomacular traction

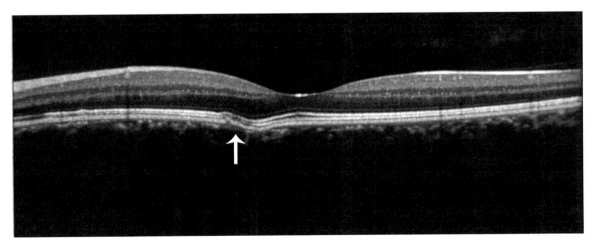

Pseudodrusen appear as small areas of elevation and reflective material above the RPE

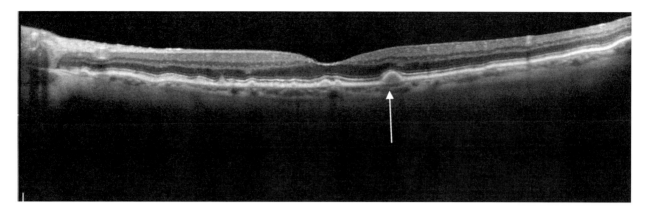

Pseudodrusen can also appear along with drusen (arrow)

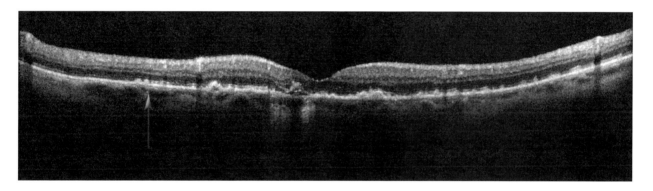

Multiple pseudodrusen

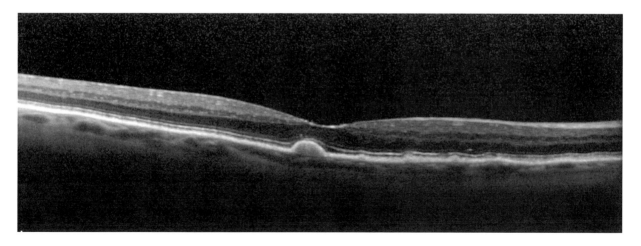

Drusen and pseudodrusen

## Age-related Macular Degeneration (AMD)

As discussed at the beginning of this chapter, AMD is one of the leading causes of blindness and is a frequent disease that is imaged in ophthalmic practices. Pigment Epithelial Detachment, (PED), is frequently found on OCT in patients with wet AMD. With the advent of new treatments for exudative, or wet AMD, OCT imaging has played a large role in the clinical decision making for physicians.

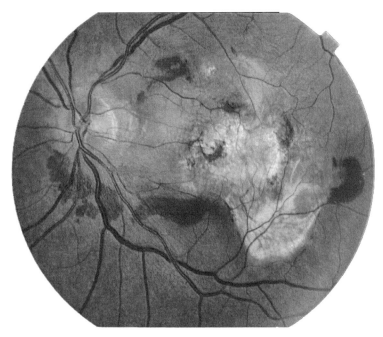

**Color fundus photograph of a patient with exudative AMD**

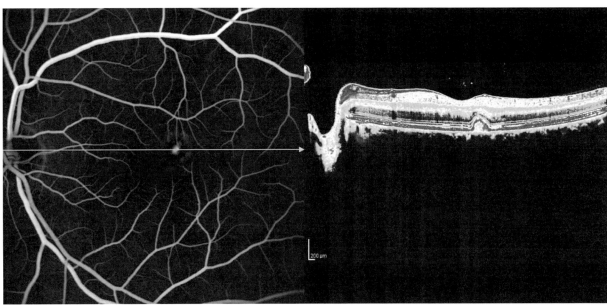

**Fluorescein angiogram with hyperfluorescence corresponding to RPE detachment seen on OCT**

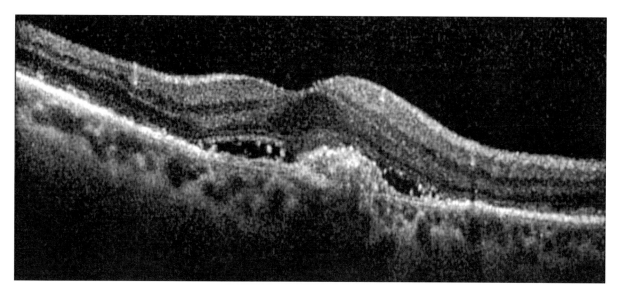

Sub retinal fluid with large hyper reflective area under the RPE

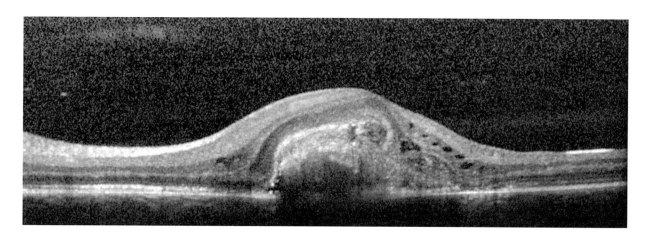

Large PED with multiple areas of intraretinal fluid

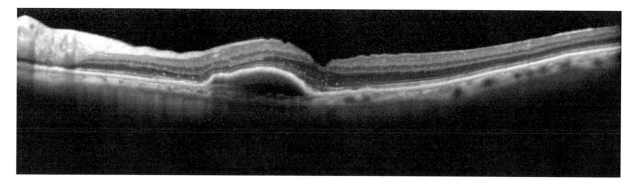

PED with no fluid in sub retinal space

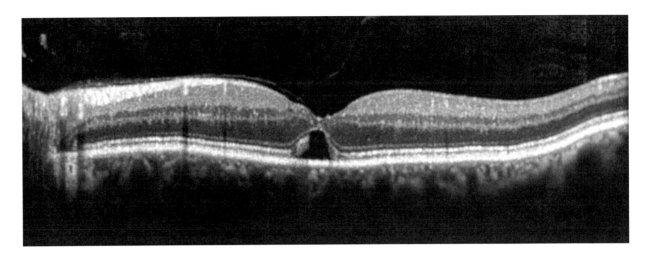

PED with intact Bruch's Membrane

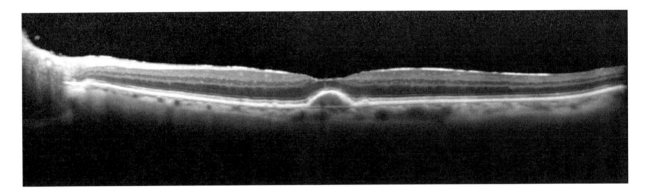

Subfoveal PED

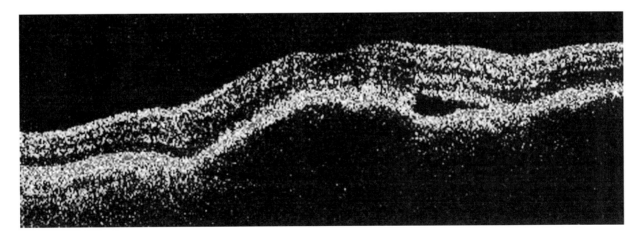

Large PED with sub retinal fluid on Time Domain OCT

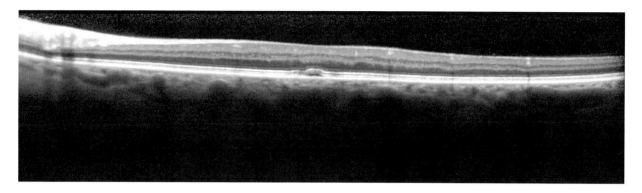

Small PED outside of the foveal (note the absence of a foveal depression)

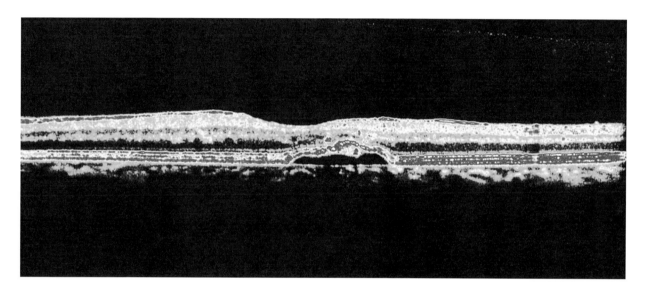

PED with fairly intact Bruch's Membrane

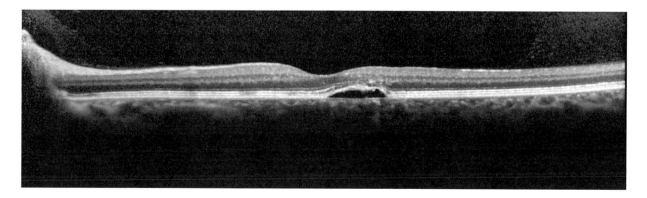

PED with no elevation of the fovea

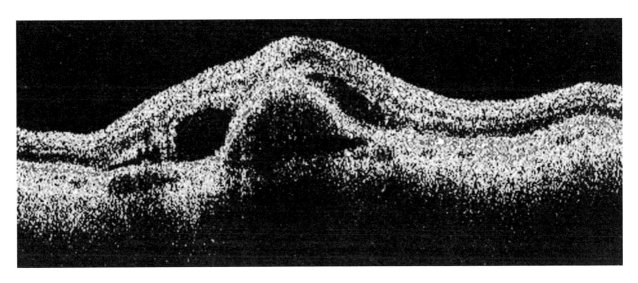

Large PED with sub retinal fluid "buttresses" on Time Domain OCT

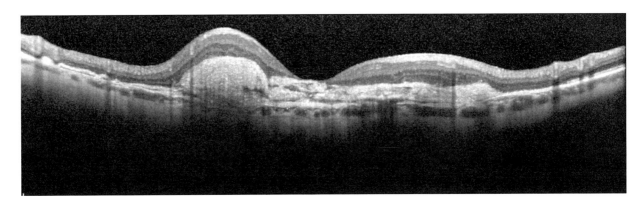

Large sub foveal scar extending throughout the macula

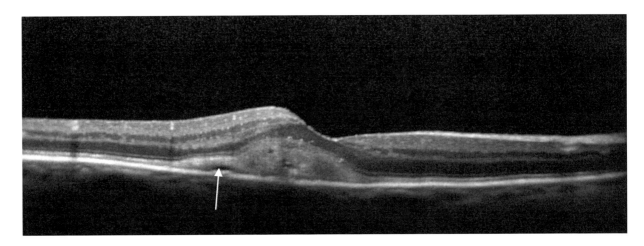

Sub foveal scar with minimal sub RPE fluid temporally (arrow)

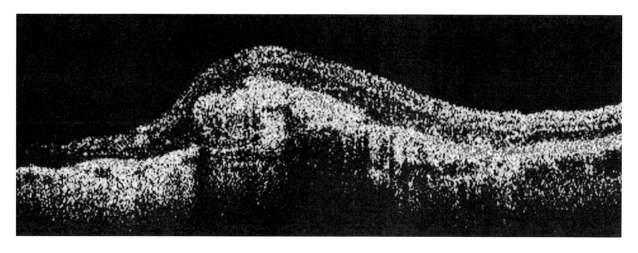

Time domain OCT of PED and scarring

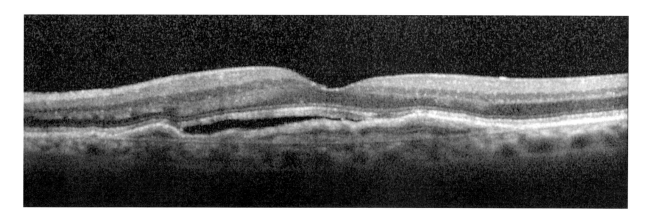

Horizontal scan showing sub retinal fluid

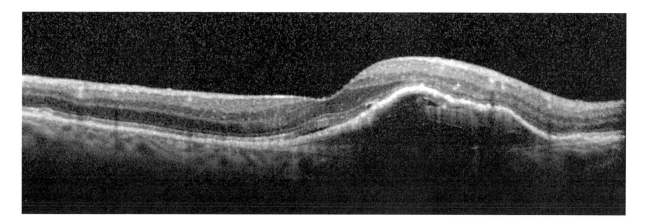

Vertical scan of same eye as above showing PED

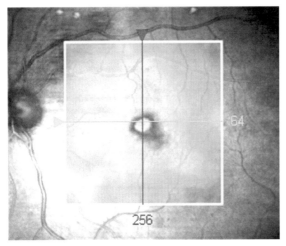 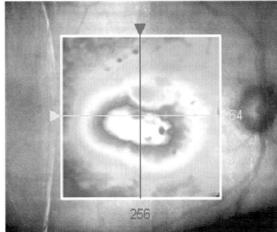

Volumetric OCT of bilateral PED

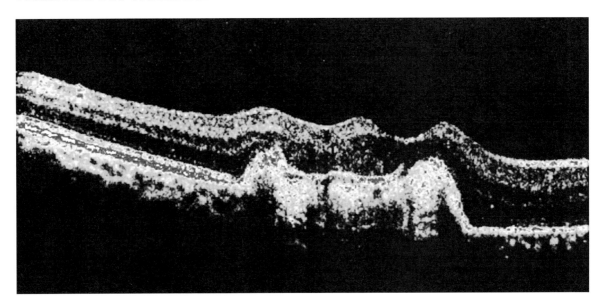

Spectral Domain scan of sub retinal scar.  Note the hyper reflectivity of the scar

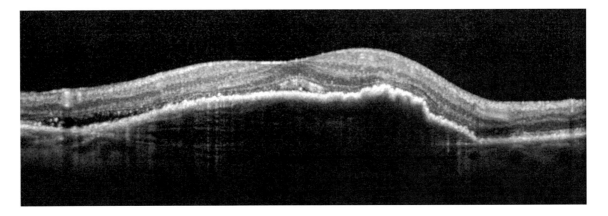

Large PED with some sub retinal fluid

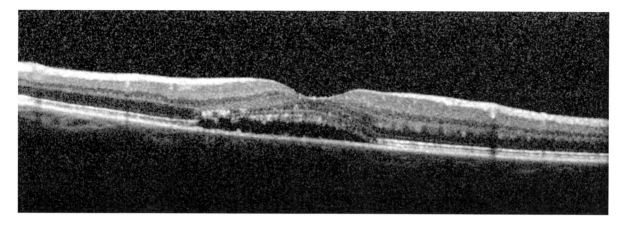

**Sub retinal fluid**

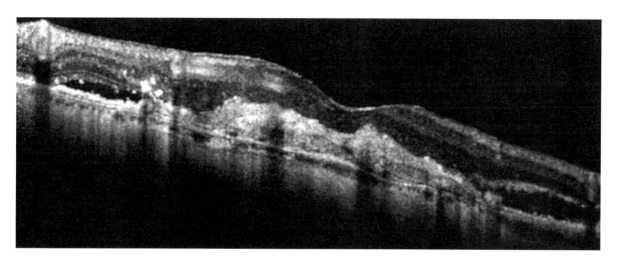

**Large sub foveal fibrovascular scar with sub retinal fluid**

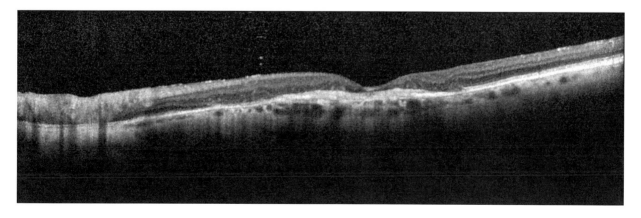

**Sub foveal fibrovascular scar**

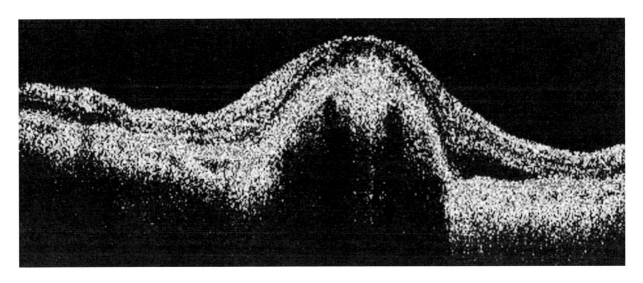

Large PED with sub retinal fluid on Time Domain OCT

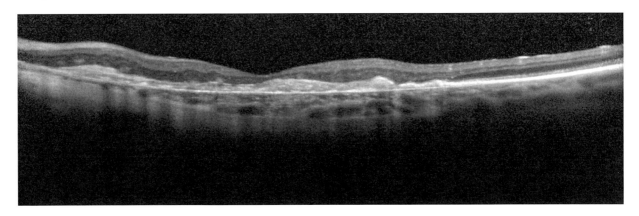

Large area of fibrovascular scar extending throughout the macula

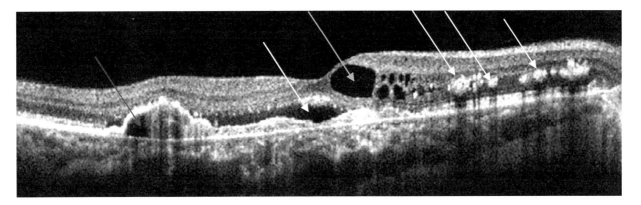

Fibrovascular scar with sub RPE fluid (red arrow) sub retinal fluid (white arrow), intraretinal fluid (green arrow) and lipid exudates (yellow arrows)

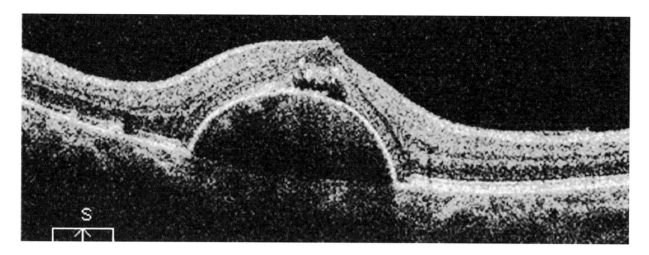

Large PED with slight sub retinal fluid

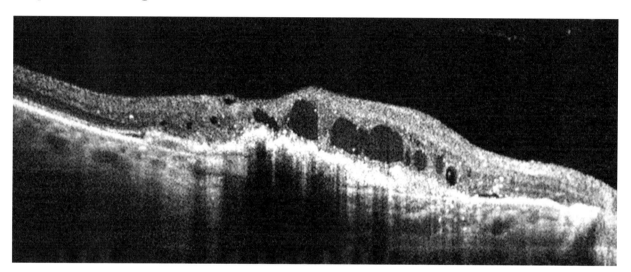

Large PED and fibrovascular scar with intraretinal fluid

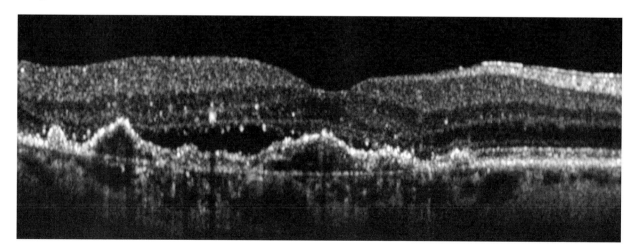

Multiple PED and sub retinal fluid

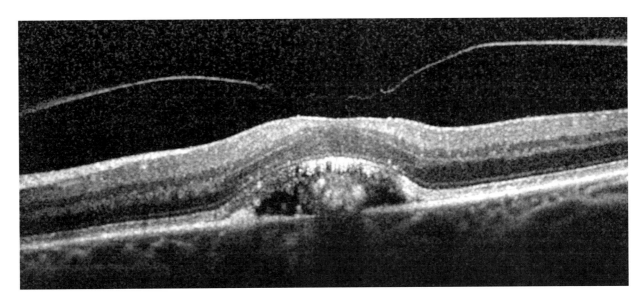

**Sub RPE fluid with hyper reflective material (cnv or scar)**

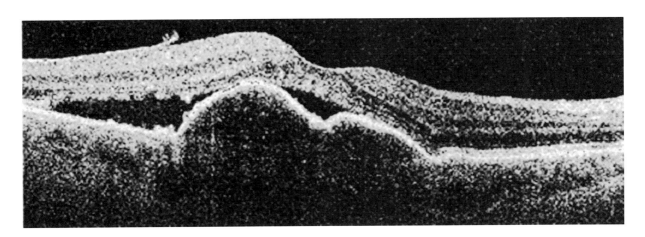

**RPE detachment with sub retinal fluid**

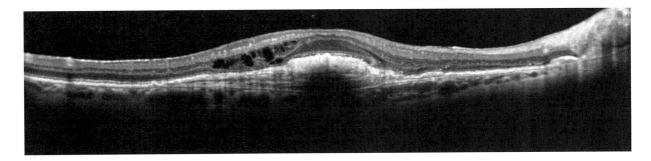

**PED with intraretinal fluid**

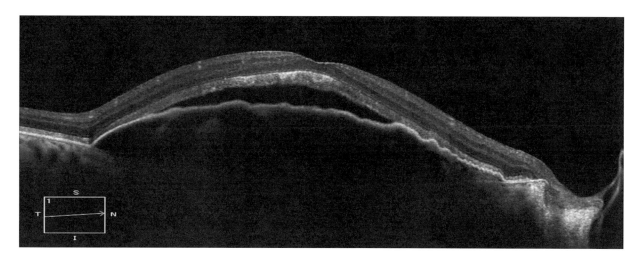

Very large PED with sub retinal fluid

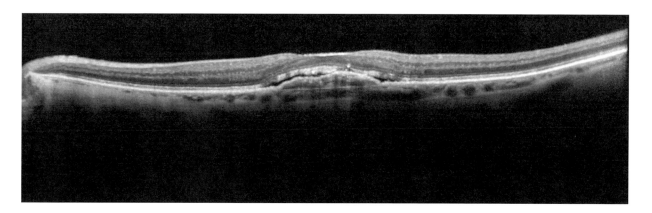

Trace sub retinal fluid with sub RPE hyper reflectivity (possibly a fibrovascular scar)

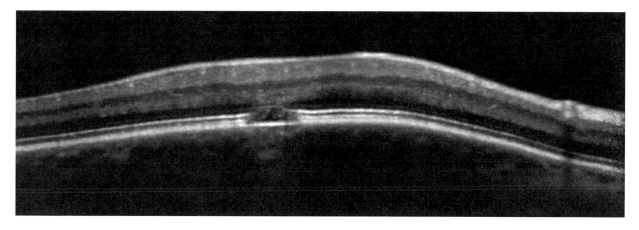

Disruption of RPE and photoreceptor cell layer. Image is taken outside of the fovea, hence the absence of a foveal depression

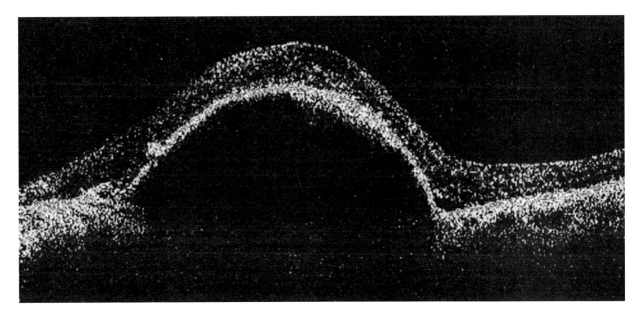

Large PED with trace sub retinal fluid on Time Domain OCT

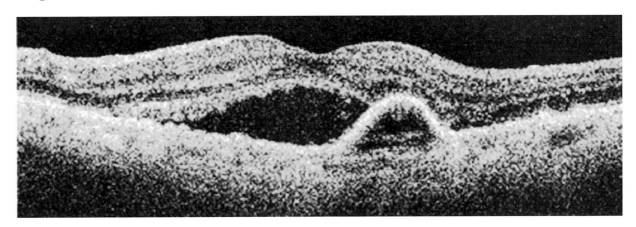

RPE detachment with sub retinal fluid

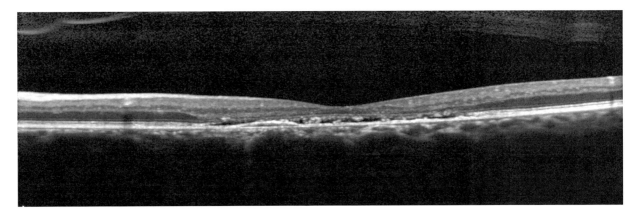

Trace sub retinal fluid

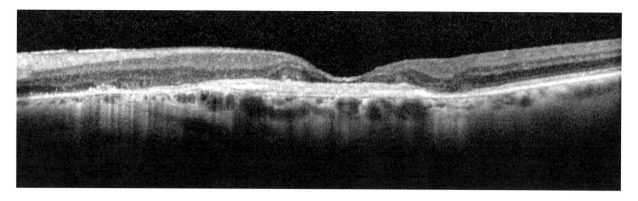

Sub foveal fibrovascular scar

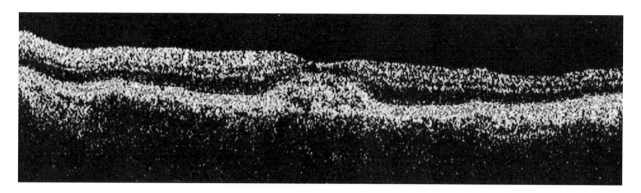

Sub foveal fibrovascular scar on Time Domain

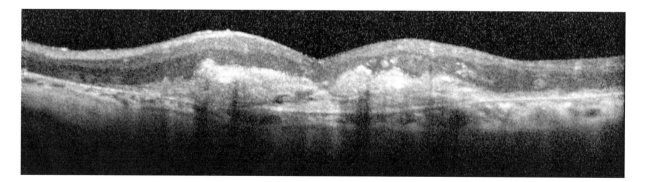

Large fibrovascular scar

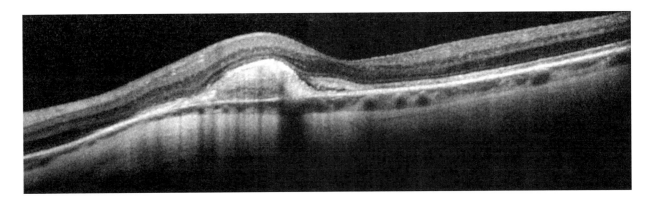

Large fibrovascular scar inferior to fovea

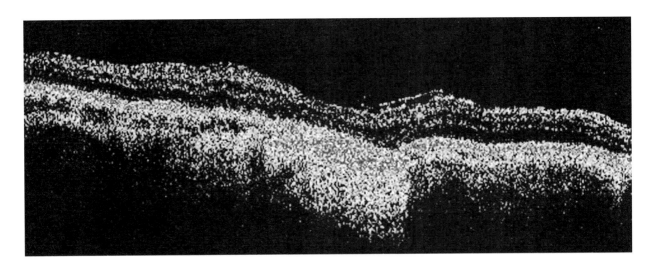

Dense sub foveal fibrovascular scar on Time Domain OCT

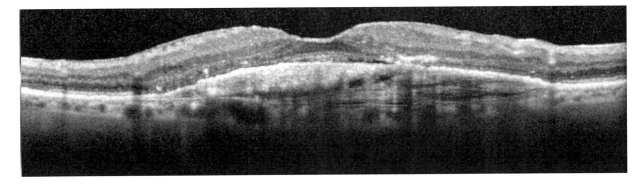

Large fibrovascular scar under the RPE

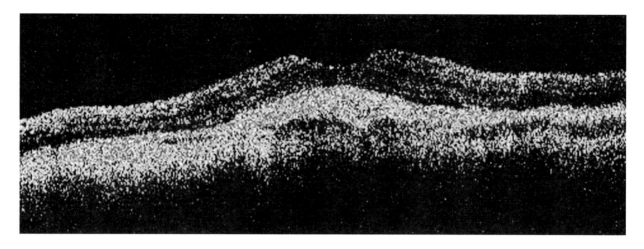

Fibrovascular scar on Time Domain OCT

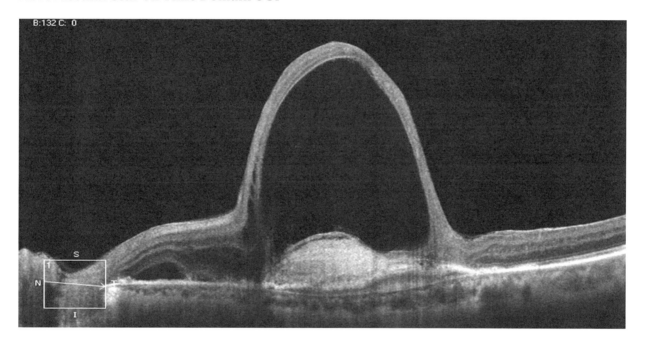

Very large area of sub retinal fluid with fibrovascular scar at the level of the RPE

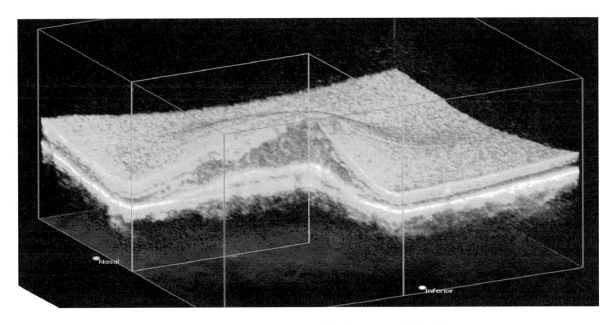

**Three-dimensional view of a large pocket of sub retinal fluid**

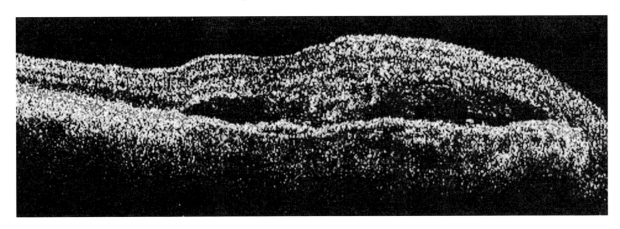

**Sub retinal fluid on Time Domain OCT**

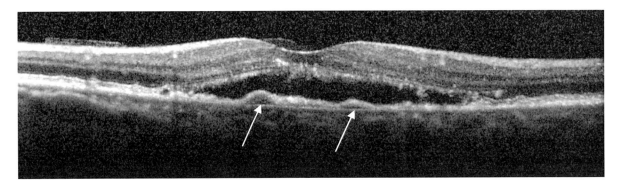

**Sub retinal fluid with intact RPE, and possibly small RPE detachments (arrows)**

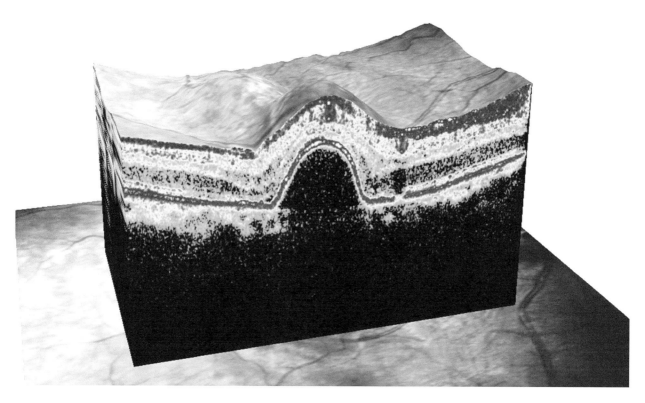

Three dimensional view of a PED

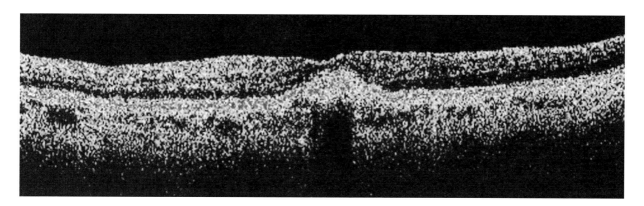

Foveal scar on Time Domain OCT. Note the absence of signal below the scar

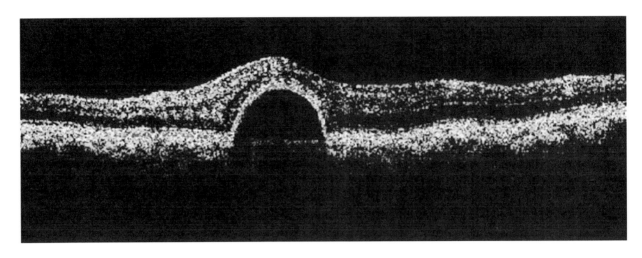

PED on Time Domain OCT. Note the faint line of Bruch's Membrane

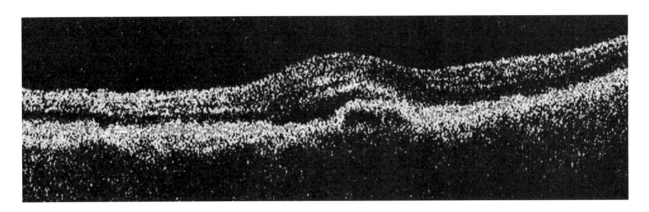

PED with sub retinal fluid on Time Domain OCT

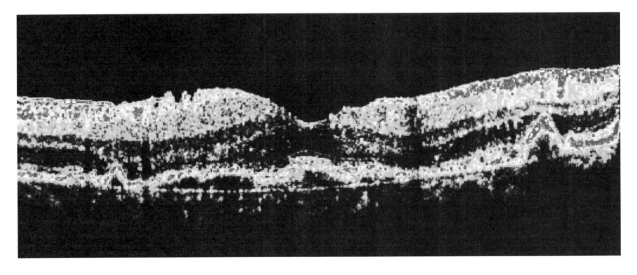

Multiple PED. Note the distinct line of Bruch's Membrane

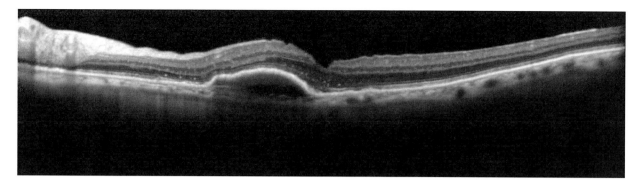

PED with hyper reflectivity in the intraretinal layer

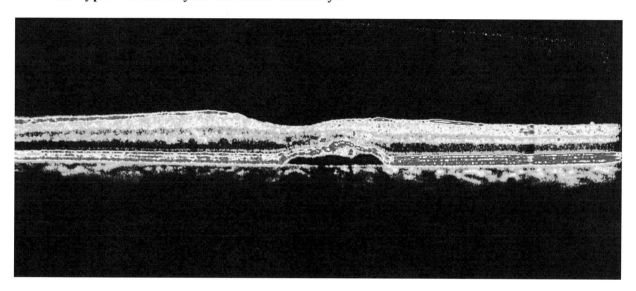

PED on Spectral Domain

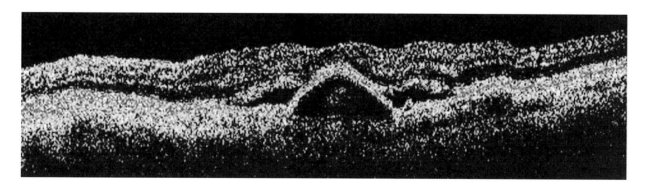

PED with sub retinal buttresses of fluid

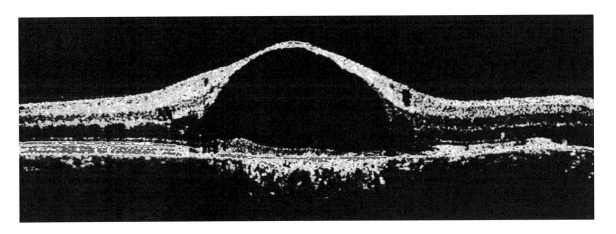

Large pocket of sub retinal fluid with intact RPE

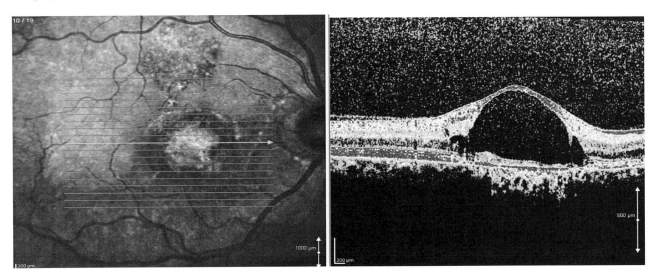

Raster scan using multiple scans to acquire a volumetric measurement (above and below)

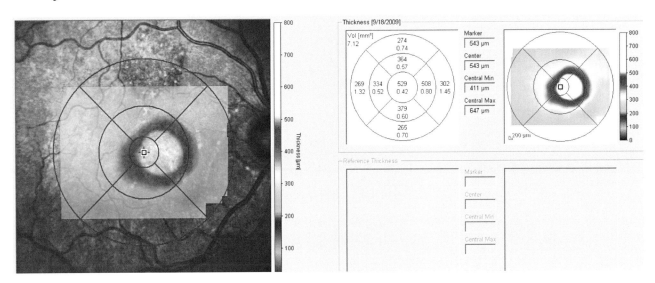

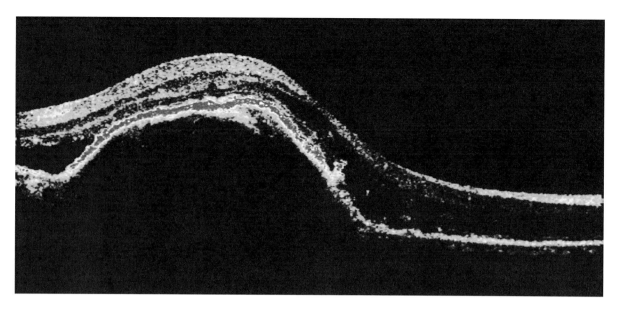

**Very large PED with sub retinal fluid**

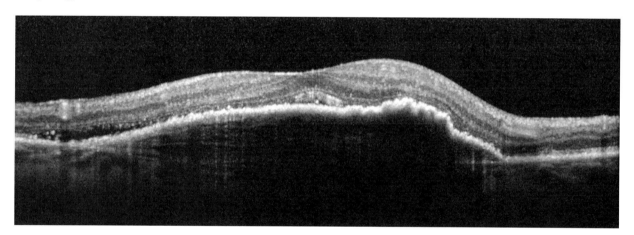

**Large PED**

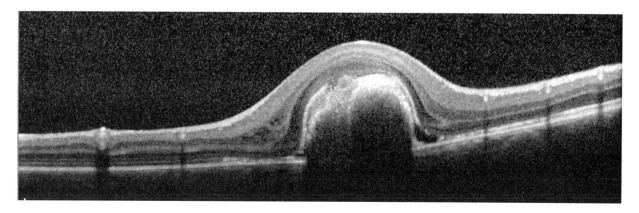

**PED. Note absence of foveal depression due to elevated retinal tissue from the PED**

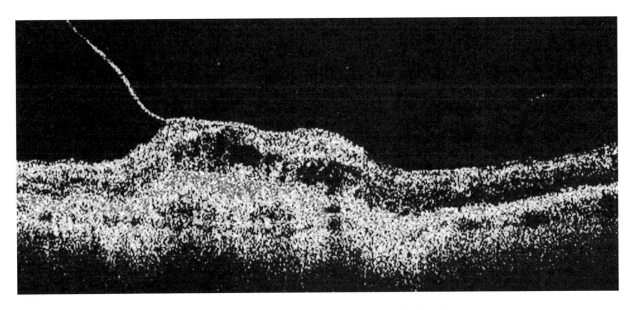

Vitreomacular traction, sub retinal scar and sub retinal fluid

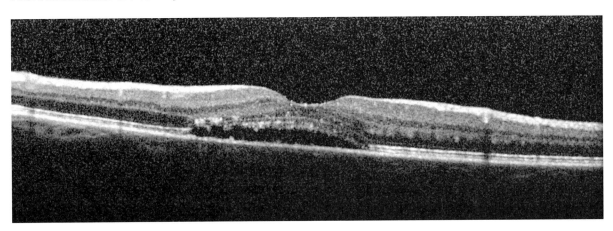

Sub retinal fluid

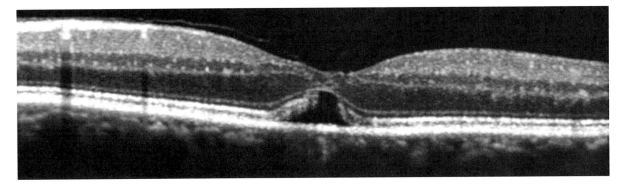

Enlarged view of a PED with separation of the RPE. Note the intact line above the RPE separation, representing either photoreceptor layer or external limiting membrane

128

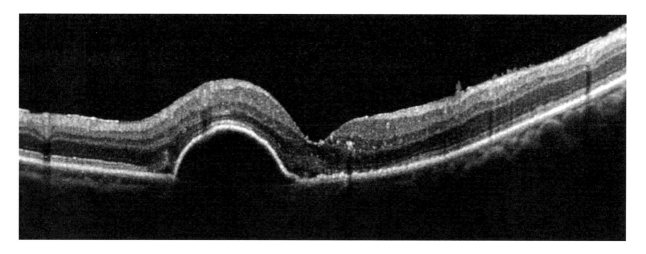

**PED temporal to the fovea**

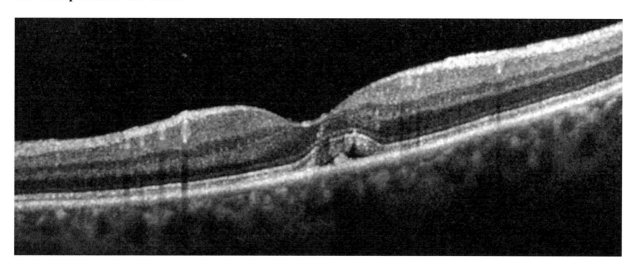

**Trace sub RPE fluid with hyper reflective material under the RPE representing drusen**

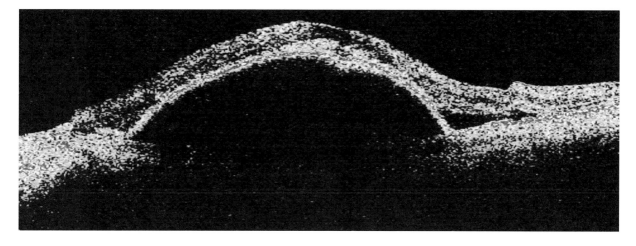

**Large PED with sub retinal fluid**

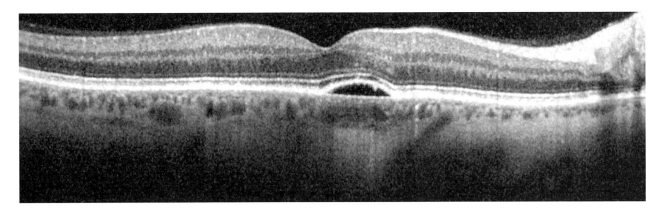

**Small PED with intact Bruch's Membrane**

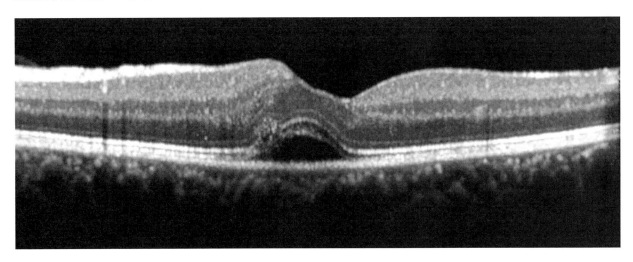

**PED with intact Bruch's Membrane**

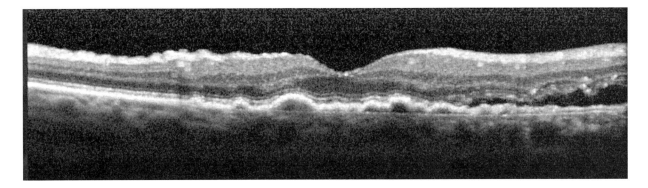

**Multiple RPE detachments with sub retinal fluid**

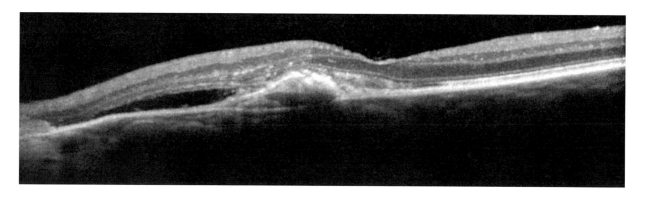

**Small PED with sub retinal fluid**

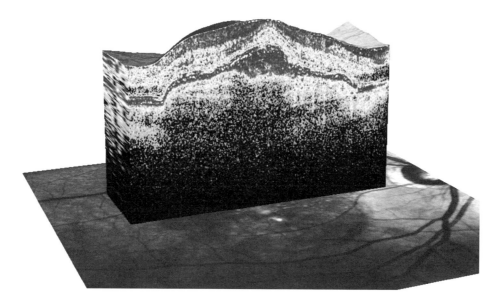

**3D cube OCT of PED and Subfoveal scar**

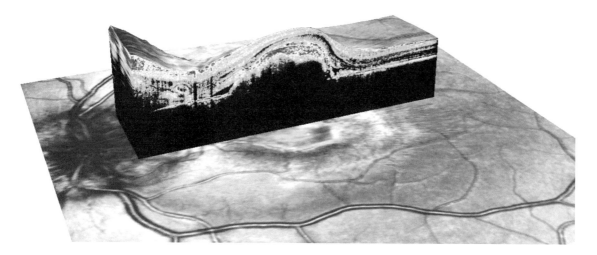

**3D Cube OCT of a PED**

# Central Serous Retinopathy (CSR)

Central Serous Retinopathy is a chorioretinal disease that is characterized by a neurosensory retinal detachment with or without a retinal pigment epithelial detachment. Although termed retinopathy, it is more appropriately designated a choroidopathy. The typical CSR patient is between 20 and 50 years old, and it affects men 6 times more than women. CSR has also been associated with stress, and is quite common in patients with "Type A" personalities. CSR is usually self-limiting, and tends to clear within 8 weeks, with recovery of vision in approximately 90% of patients. [35]

Patients typically present with complaints of metamorphopsia and may complain of blurriness. In patients over the age of 50, CSR may be indistinguishable from exudative macular degeneration, although AMD may present with both hemorrhagic neurosensory retinal detachment and hemorrhagic RPE detachments. [36]

On OCT, central serous retinopathy presents with an area of fluid in the sub retinal space, between the neurosensory retina and the retinal pigment epithelium. In the author's experience, a large portion of CSR patients do not present with complete retinal pigment epithelial detachments, instead the RPE is largely intact. In some of the examples here, the RPE has reflective tissue on the surface, which may represent a splitting of the RPE or depositing of remnants of the RPE on the anterior surface of Bruch's Membrane, with a "stalactite" appearance of the RPE on the posterior surface of the neurosensory retina.

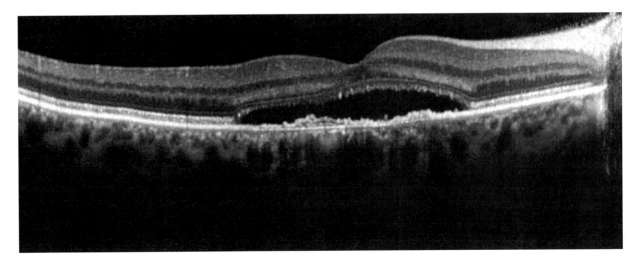

**Note the sub retinal fluid under the fovea, with intact RPE**

132

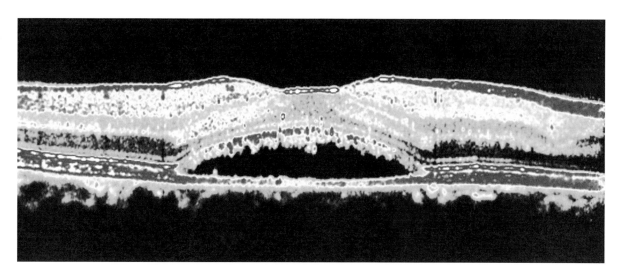

Typical "stalactite" formation at the roof of the sub retinal detachment

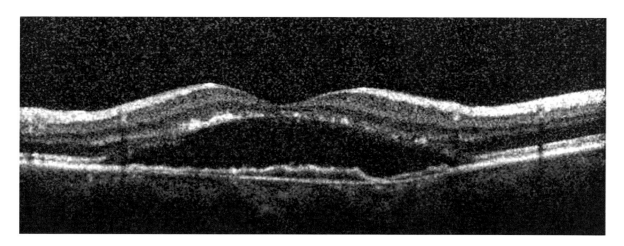

Sub retinal fluid with slight elevation of the RPE

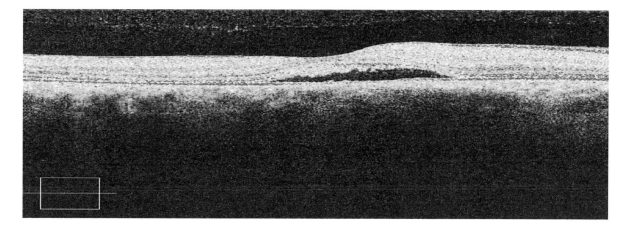

Atypical CSR with elevated PED

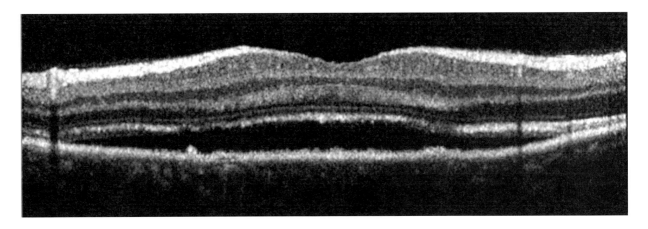

CSR with separation of the RPE

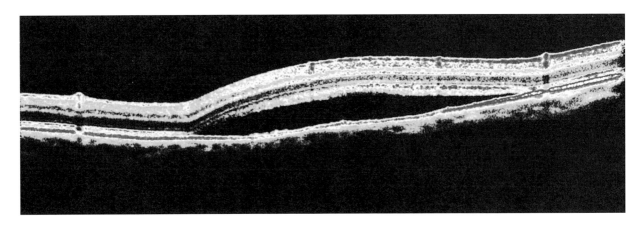

Similar "splitting' of the RPE

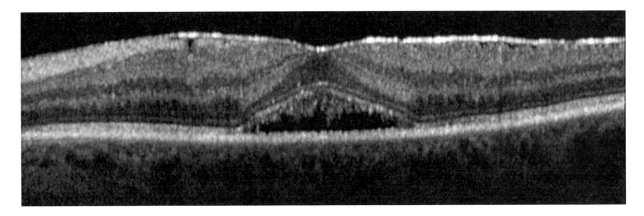

CSR with stalactite type formation on the posterior surface of the neurosensory retina

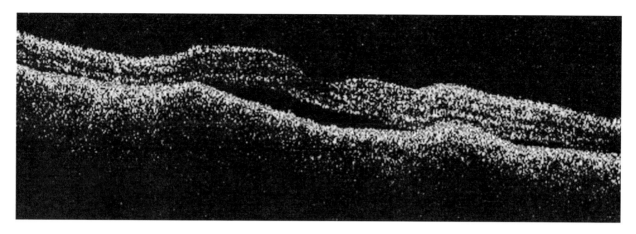

**CSR with sub retinal fluid**

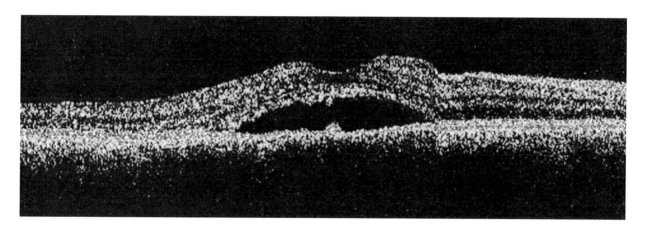

**Typical "stalactite" formation in CSR**

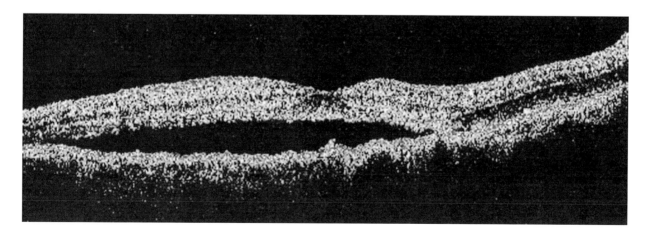

**Large area of sub retinal fluid**

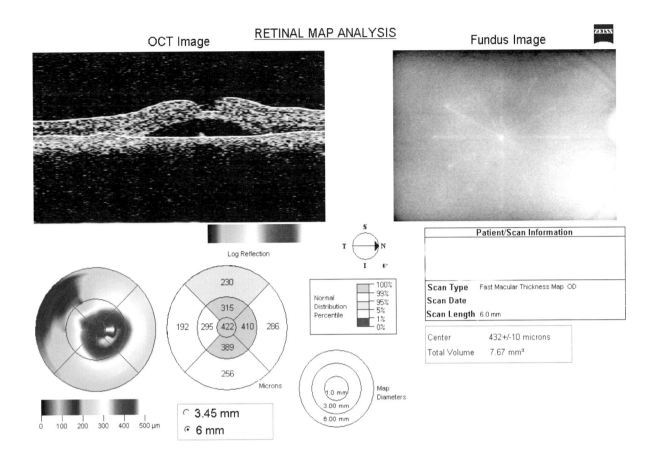

**Volumetric OCT from a radial pattern scan**

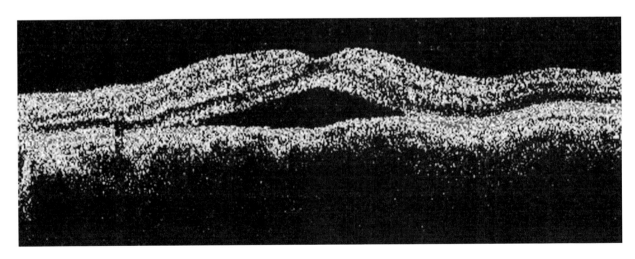

**Time Domain OCT with possible RPE detachment vs. sub retinal fluid**

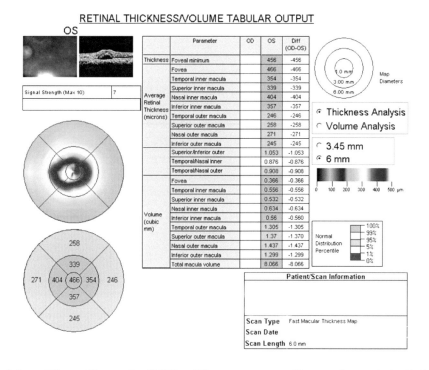

**Sub retinal fluid on Time Domain OCT with corresponding volumetric/tabular OCT**

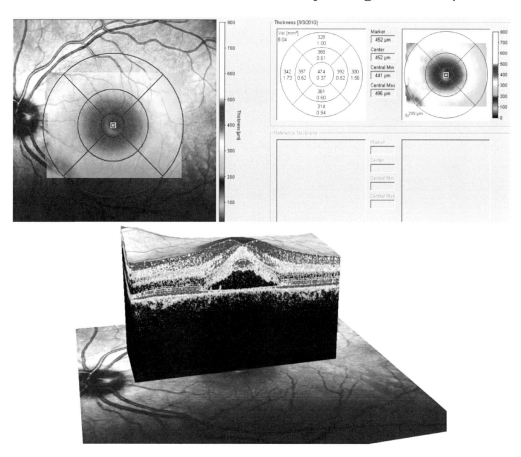

**Volumetric OCT (top) and 3D cube OCT of CSR**

## Retinal Angiomotous Proliferation (RAP)

The term RAP describes a distinct form of occult choroidal neovascularization associated with proliferation of intraretinal capillaries in the macular area that proliferates into the sub retinal space. [36]

RAP was first recognized and described in 1992 as a deep retinal vascular anomalous complex. [37] In 2000, another group noted the presence of retinal-choroidal anastomosis in RAP, but emphasized that this variant can occur without the presence of pigment epithelial detachments. [38]

RAP is difficult to image solely with OCT, as angiography, specifically Indocyanine Green Angiography (ICG), is usually needed to direct the OCT scan.

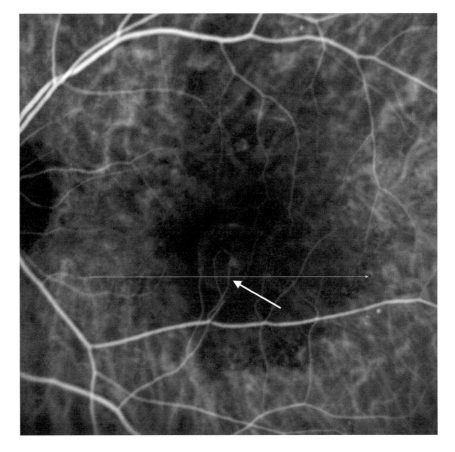

**Fluorescein angiogram of RAP lesion with perforating retinal vessel indicated by arrow**

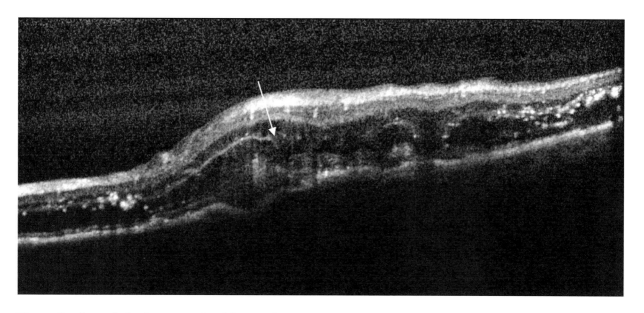

Note the break in intraretinal boundary (arrow) where the retinal vessel leads to neovascular membrane

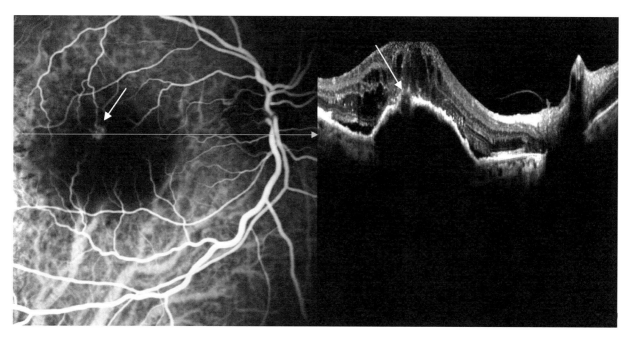

Angiography directed OCT reveals a break in RPE corresponding with the retinal vessel illustrated on angiography

## Geographic Atrophy

Geographic Atrophy (GA) is characterized by one or more well defined, usually more or less circular, patches of partial or complete depigmentation of the retinal pigment epithelium, typically with exposure of underlying large choroidal blood vessels. End stage dry macular degeneration can result in geographic atrophy, and there are no available effective treatments to arrest the progression of GA, which often results in significant central vision loss. 43 On OCT atrophy presents as a hyper reflective pattern under the RPE and in some cases, neurosensory retina may be thinned to the level of the RPE.

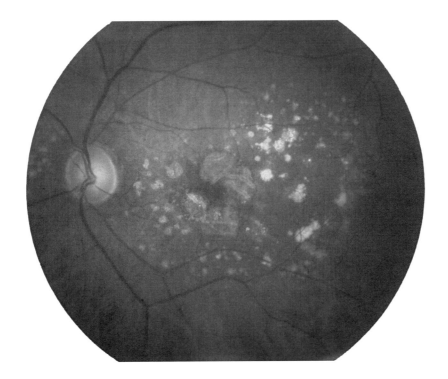

**Color fundus photograph of geographic atrophy**

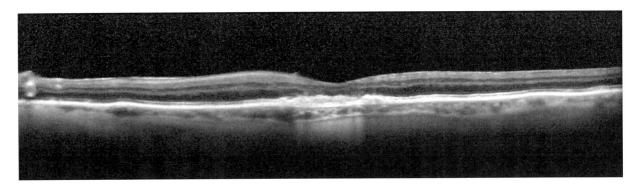

**Hyper reflectivity under the fovea indicates an area of geographic atrophy**

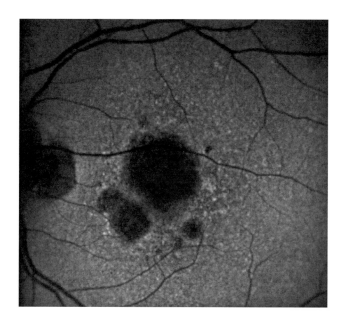

Geographic atrophy represented by dark areas on autofluorescent imaging

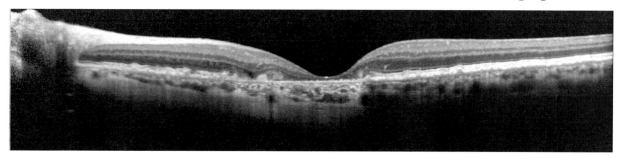

Note the thinning of neurosensory retina in the fovea and absence of photoreceptor cell layer

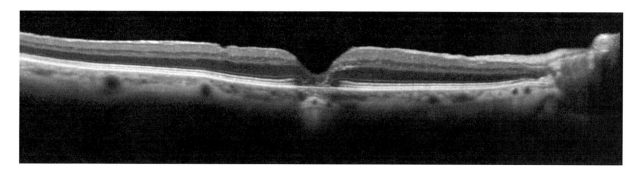

Thinning neurosensory retina

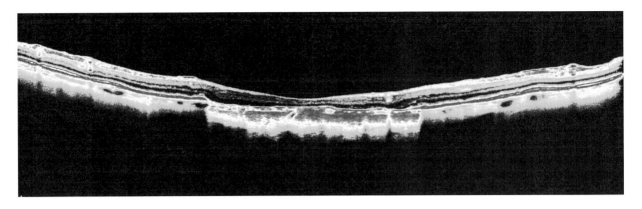

Large area of hyper reflective geographic atrophy under the macula

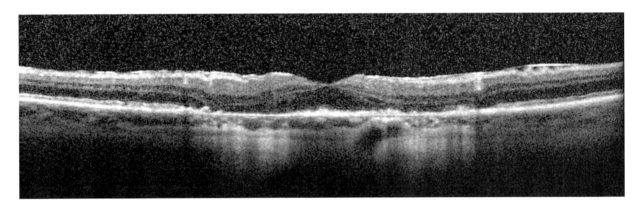

Hyper reflective areas under the fovea showing geographic atrophy

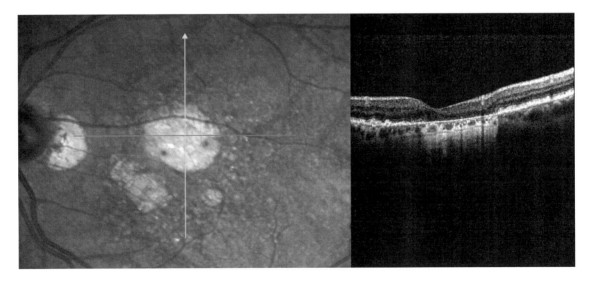

Fundus image on left, with geographic atrophy patches in white. Corresponding vertical OCT scan on right

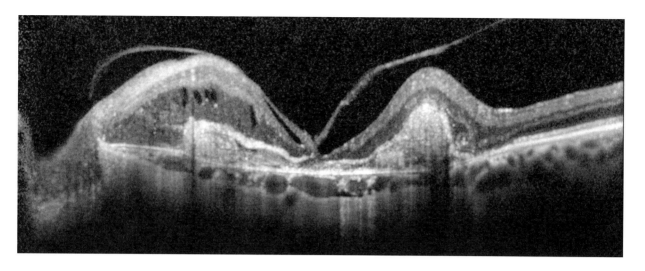

Geographic atrophy with vitreomacular traction, sub retinal scar, and intraretinal fluid

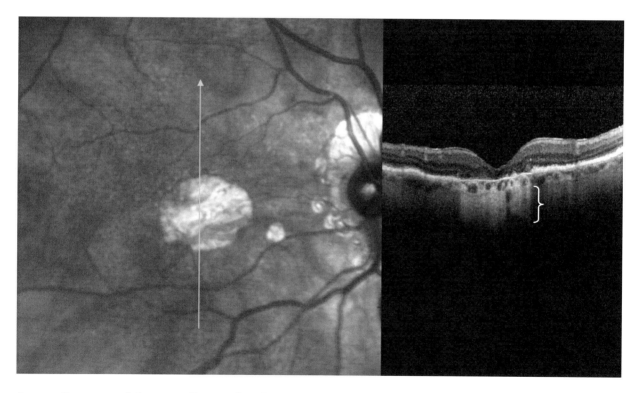

Area of geographic atrophy on fundus image and corresponding OCT scan

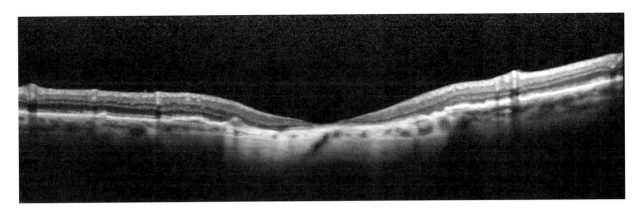

Large area of geographic atrophy and thinning neurosensory retina in the fovea

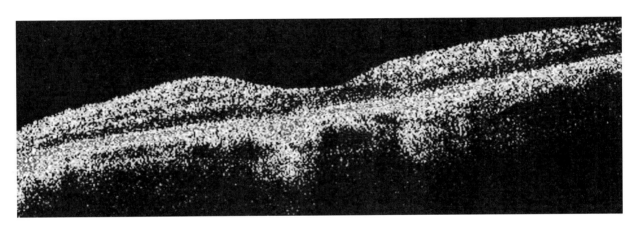

Time Domain OCT image of geographic atrophy

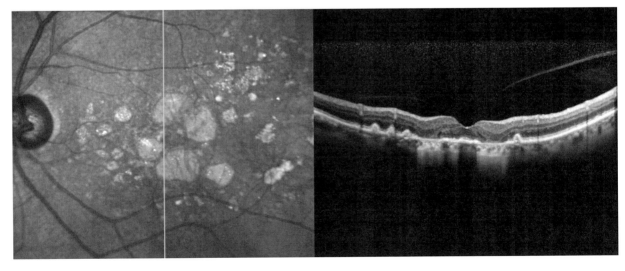

Multiple areas of geographic atrophy. Note the hyper reflective areas on either side of the fovea, corresponding with the two areas of atrophy inferiorly and superiorly

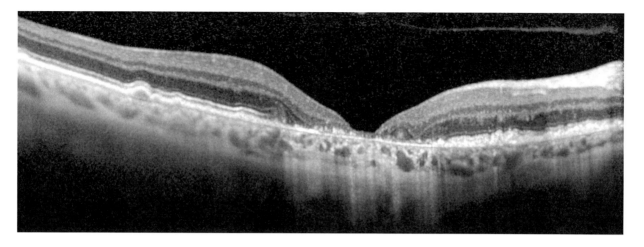

Thinning of the fovea and absence of the photoreceptor cell layer

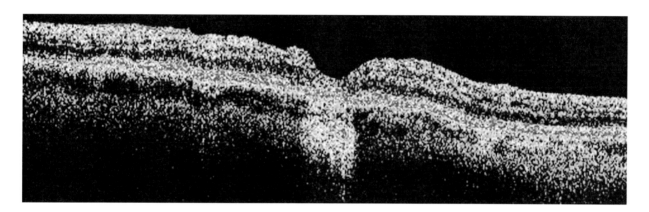

Time Domain OCT with thinning of the fovea and hyper reflective area under the fovea

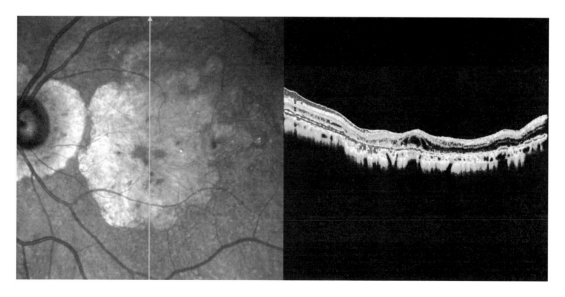

# Choroid

The choroid is the layer beneath Bruch's Membrane, and is made up of blood vessels primarily responsible for the diffusion of metabolites to and from the RPE and the outer half of the retina. The choriocapillaris contains some of the largest capillaries in the body, with some under the macula that are up to 20 microns in diameter. [41]

Somewhat easier to image the choroid with Spectral Domain OCT, the choroid can be difficult to image with Time Domain OCT. The multiple layers of retina, especially the RPE, that reflect light back to the OCT system decreases the intensity and reflectance signal of the light by the time it reaches the choroid. One method to image the choroid better is called enhanced depth imaging OCT. At this time, the literature describing the technique involves moving the OCT head closer to the eye, therefore inverting the OCT image seen by the technician, and providing a better view of the choroidal structures. The image is then inverted back to a more recognizable orientation, using peripheral software. This technique has allowed clinicians to determine the thickness of the choroid as well as the absence of choroidal vessels under the macula. [42]

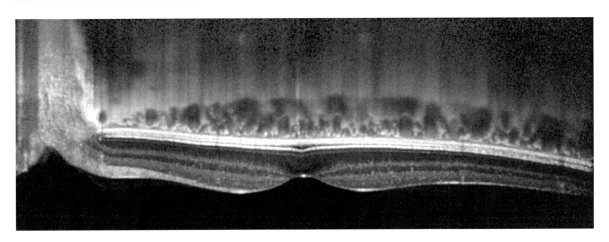

**Inverted OCT image**

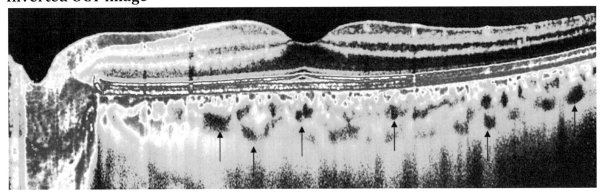

**Re-inverted OCT scan illustrating normal choroidal thickness. Note the large choroidal vessels (arrows)**

146

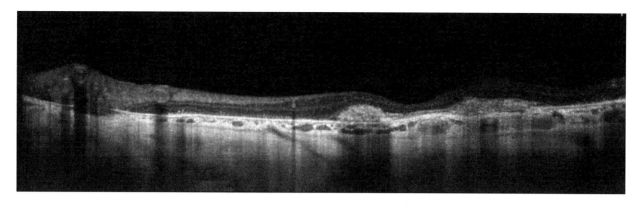

Thinning of choroid. Note the absence of many large choroidal vessels under the macula

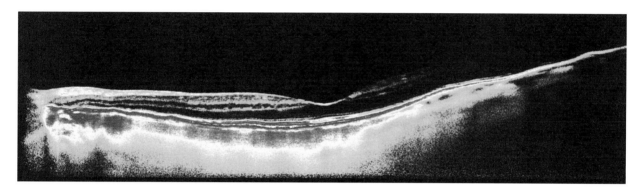

Thin choroid with absence of choroidal vessels

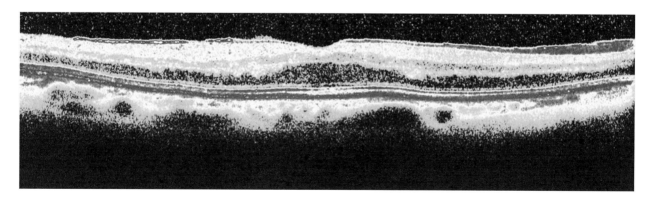

Note thin choroid with only a few choroidal vessels

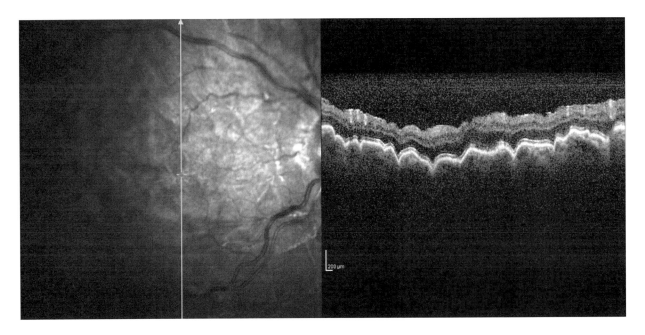

**Choroidal Folds**

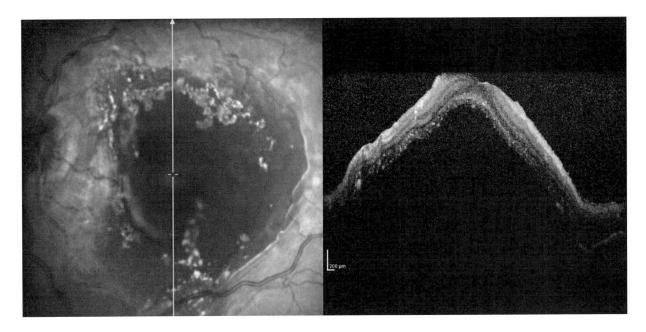

**Choroidal Hemorrhage**

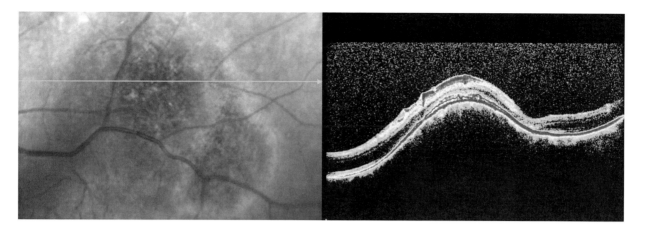

Choroidal Melanoma

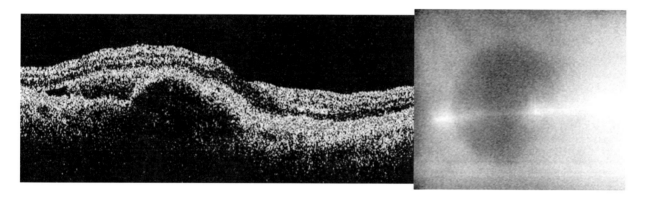

Choroidal Melanoma on Time Domain OCT

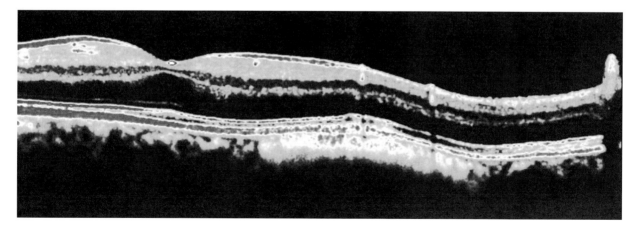

Dense reflectivity sub RPE indicates hyper pigmentation of a nevus

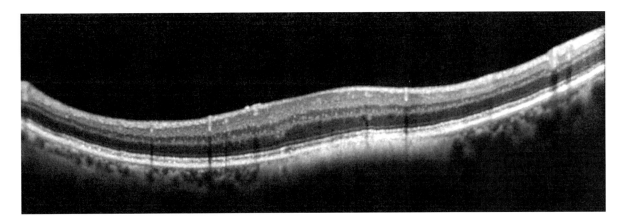

Note the absence of reflectivity in the choroid under the nevus, due to the absorption of light in the hyper pigmentation of the nevus

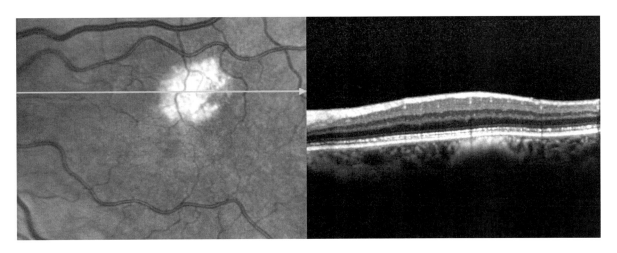

Nevus shows as a white area on infrared wavelength of light

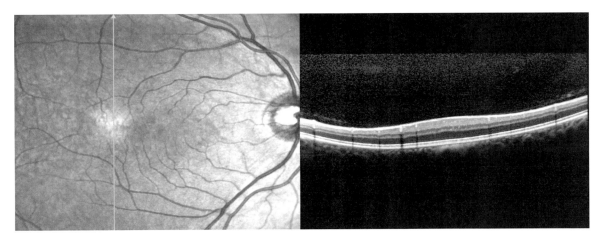

Small nevus

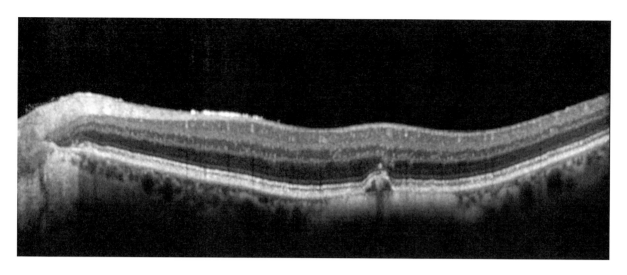

Small area of RPE disruption outside the fovea

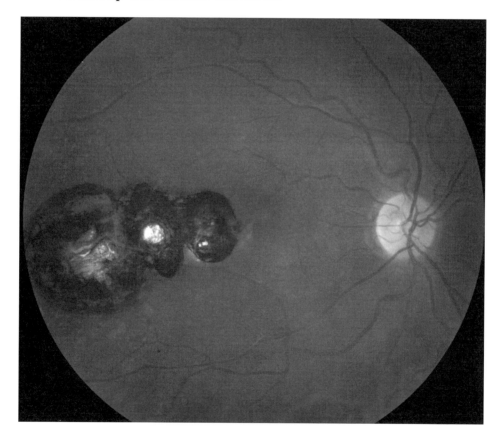

Color fundus image of congenital hypertrophy of the retinal pigment epithelium (CHRPE)

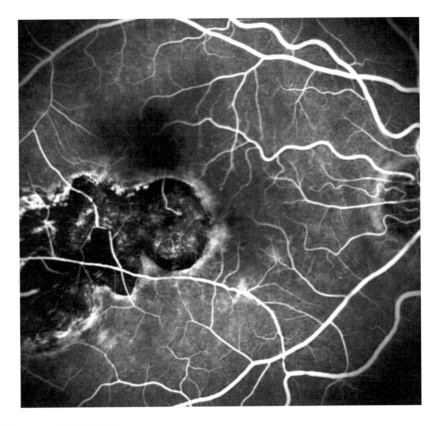

**Fluorescein image of CHRPE**

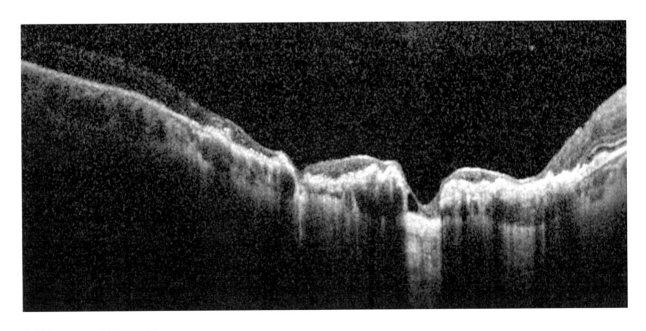

**OCT scan of CHRPE**

# D. Other Retinal Pathology

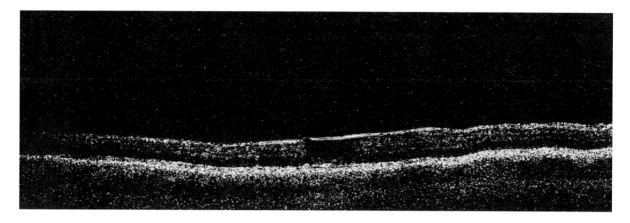

Because of the density of silicone oil, imaging on OCT can be difficult, and the interface of silicone oil and retina is highly reflective, sometimes blocking anatomy

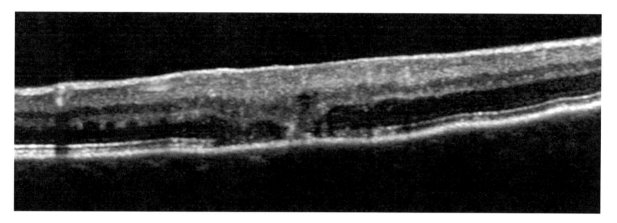

Juxtafoveal telangiectasia

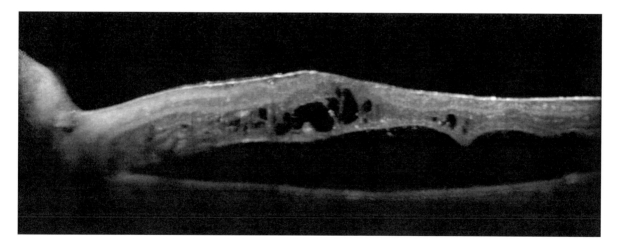

Retinal detachment with intraretinal fluid

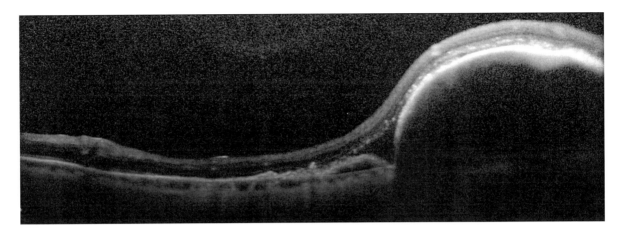

**Localized retinal detachment**

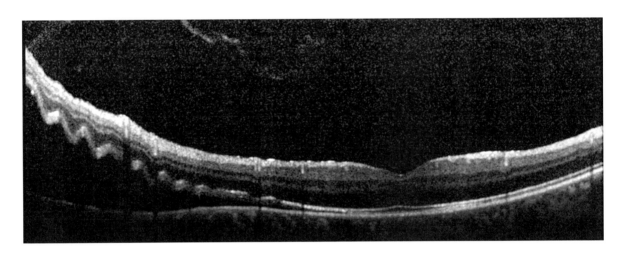

**Peripheral retinal detachment**

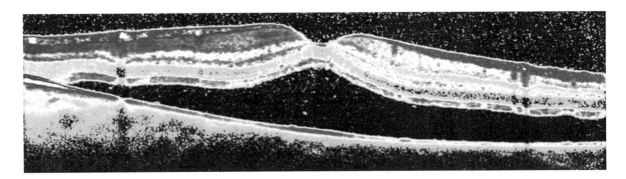

**Chronic retinal detachment**

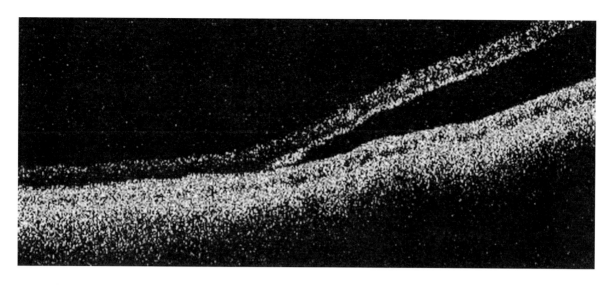

Peripheral retinal detachment on Time Domain OCT

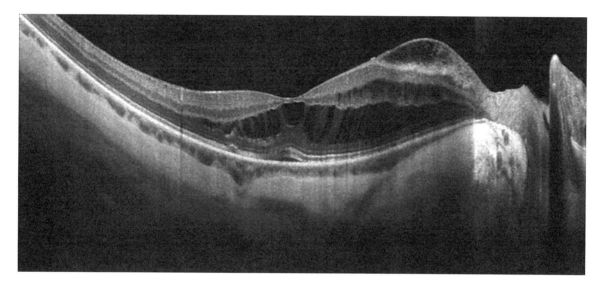

Retinoschesis. Note the separation of retinal layers and attachment of the retina

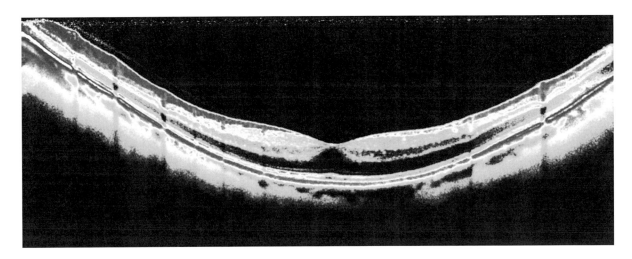

Myopic eyes will be illustrated as concave, due to the length of the eye

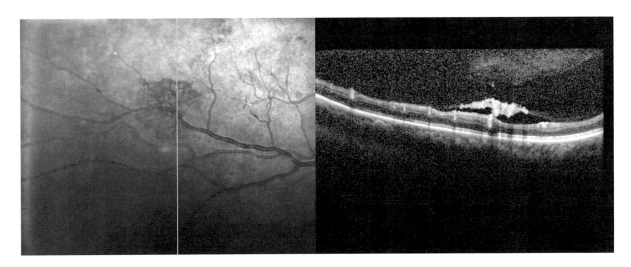

Neovascularization (NVE) in a diabetic patient

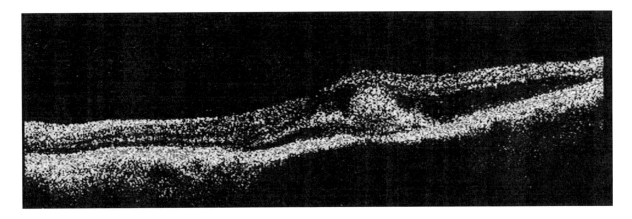

Metastatic tumor within the retina

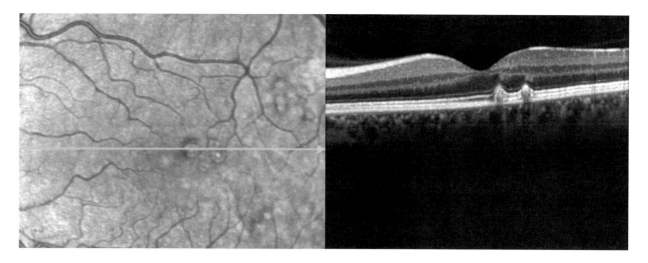

**Multifocal evanescent white dot syndrome (MEWDS)**

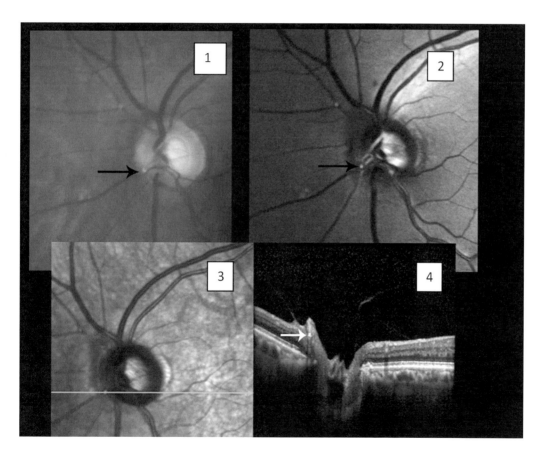

Hollenhorst plaque 1. Color fundus image 2. Red free image 3. Infrared image with OCT scan line 4. OCT image with hyper reflective plaque (arrow)

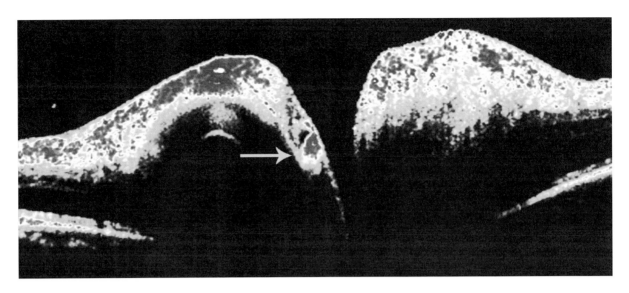

**Hollenhorst plaque on OCT (arrow)**

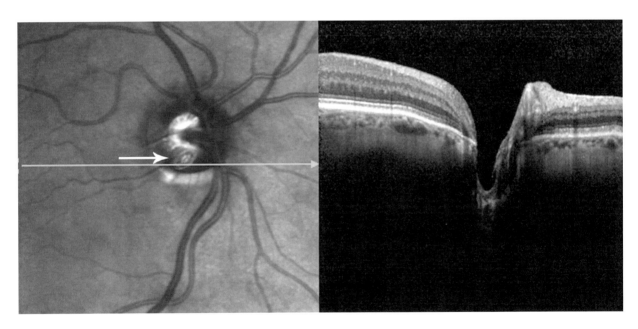

**Optic pit. Note arrow on fundus photograph indicating pit**

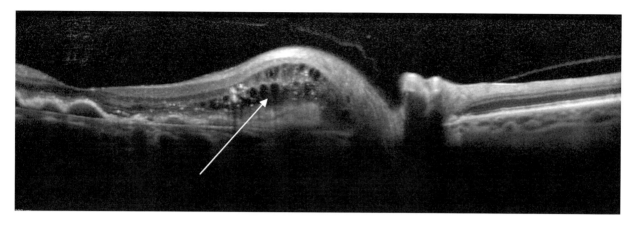

Papilledema on OCT line scan. Note the areas of edema next to the optic nerve head (arrow)

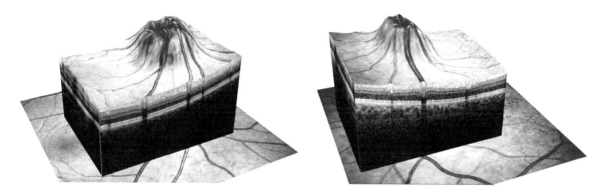

3 dimension OCT of bilateral papilledema

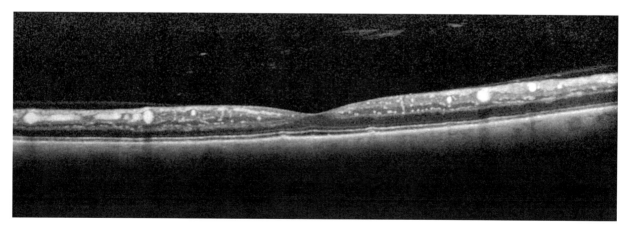

Hypercholesterolemia in retinal vessels. Note the hyper reflectance of the lipid outlining the vessels

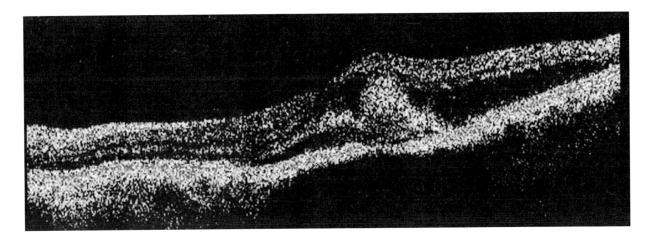

**Metastatic tumor**

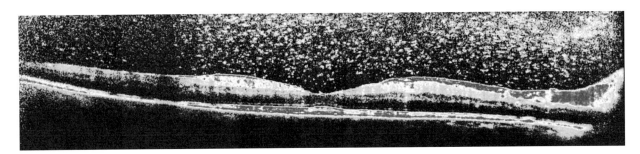

**Vitreous hemorrhage**

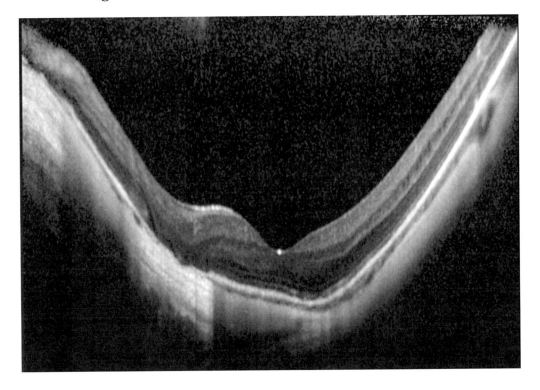

**High myope**

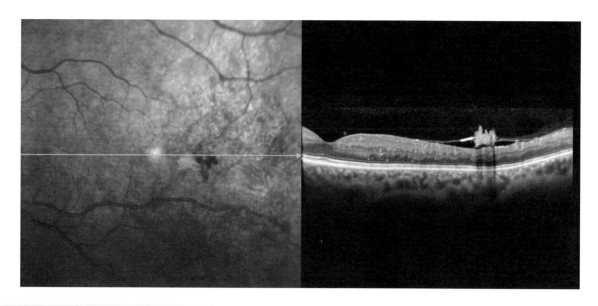

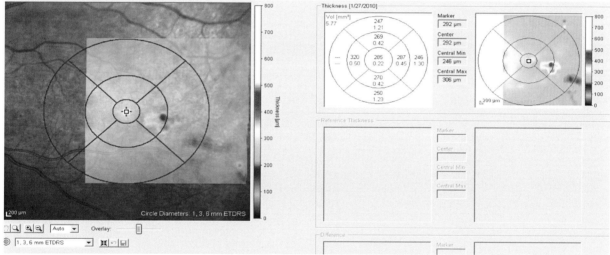

**Line scan of NVE (top) with volumetric OCT (bottom)**

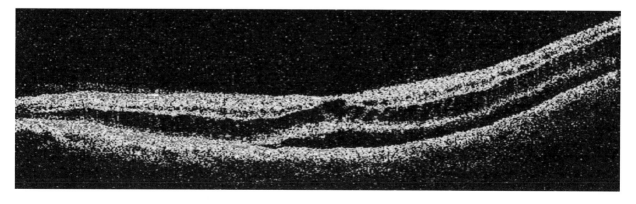

**Retinoschesis**

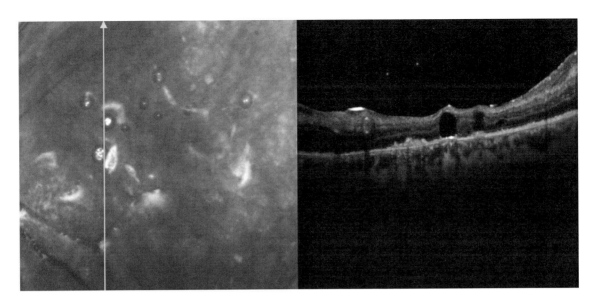

**OCT scan through perfluoron (PFO) bubbles trapped under the retina**

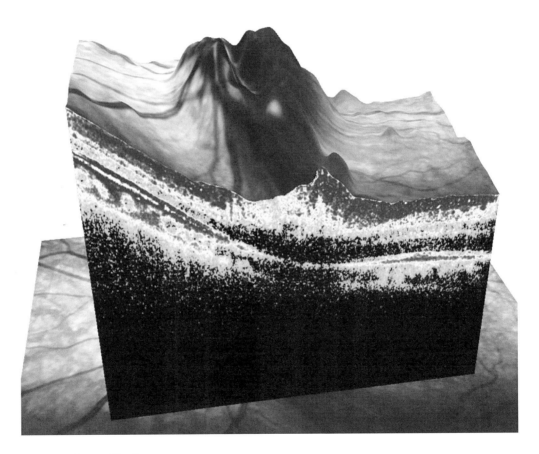

**3D cube scan of papilledema**

# V.    References

1. Huang D, Swanson EA, Lin CP, et al. Optical coherence tomography. Science 1991;254:1178-81

2. Schuman JS, Puliafito CA, Fujimoto JG. Optical Coherence Tomography of Ocular Diseases. 2nd ed. Thorofare, New Jersey: SLACK Inc., 2004

3. Schmidt-Erfurth U, Leitgeb RA, Michels S, et al. Three-dimensional ultra-high resolution of optical coherence tomography of macular disease. Invest Ophthalmol 2005;123:1715-1720

4. Schuman JS, Puliafito CA, Fujimoto JG. Optical Coherence Tomography of Ocular Diseases. 2nd ed. Thorofare, New Jersey: SLACK Inc., 2004

5. Ophthalmic Optical Coherence Tomography Market: Past, Present, & Future, Optical Coherence Tomography News, Mar 29 2009

6. Schuman JS, Puliafito CA, Fujimoto JG. Optical Coherence Tomography of Ocular Diseases. 2nd ed. Thorofare, New Jersey: SLACK Inc., 2004

7. D. Landry, *Retinal Imaging Simplified* (Bryson Taylor Publishing, 2009) p. 71

8. (Landau D, Schneidman EM, Jacobovitz T, et al: Quantitative in vivo retinal thickness measurements in healthy subjects. Ophthalmology 1997;104:639-642)

9. Regillo CD, Brown GC, Flynn HW. Vitreoretinal Disease the Essentials. Thieme Medical Publishers, Inc, 1999

10. Regillo CD, Brown GC, Flynn HW. Vitreoretinal Disease the Essentials. Thieme Medical Publishers, Inc, 1999

11. Regillo CD, Brown GC, Flynn HW. Vitreoretinal Disease the Essentials. Thieme Medical Publishers, Inc, 1999

12. Gass JDM: Stereoscopic Atlas of Macular Diseases, 4th ed., p 938. Mosby, St. Louis, 1997

13. Regillo CD, Brown GC, Flynn HW. Vitreoretinal Disease the Essentials. Thieme Medical Publishers, Inc, 1999

14. Gass JD. Lamellar hole: a complication of cystoid macular edema after cataract extraction: a clicopathologic case report. Trans Am Ophthalmol Soc 1975;73:230-250

15. Witkin et al. redefining lamellar holes and the vitreomacular interface. American Academy of Ophthalmology, 2006; 388-396, Elsevier Inc.

16. Tanner V, Chauhan DS, Jackson TL, Williamson TH. Optical coherence tomography of the vitreoretinal interface in macular hole formation. BR J Ophthalmol 2001;85:1092-1097

17. Witkin et al. redefining lamellar holes and the vitreomacular interface. American Academy of Ophthalmology, 2006; 388-396, Elsevier Inc.

18. Johnson MW, Etiology and Treatment of Macular Edema. Amer Journal of Ophthal, 7/08 11-21. Elsevier Inc.

19. Regillo CD, Brown GC, Flynn HW. Vitreoretinal Disease the Essentials. Chapter 11, 161-173. Thieme Medical Publishers, Inc, 1999

20.  Gass JDM, Norton EWD: Cystoid macular edema and papilledema following cataract extraction: a fluorescein fundoscopic and angiographic study.  Arch Ophthalmol 1966;76:646-661

21. Regillo CD, Brown GC, Flynn HW.  Vitreoretinal Disease the Essentials.  Chapter 10; Diabetic retinopathy.  Thieme Medical Publishers, Inc, 1999

22. Bolz M, Schmidt-Erfurth U, Deak G, et al, Diabetic Retinopathy Research Group Vienna.  Optical coherence tomographic hyperreflective foci: a morphologic sign of lipid extravasation in diabetic macular edema.  Ophthalmology 2009;116:914-920

23. Regillo CD, Brown GC, Flynn HW.  Vitreoretinal Disease the Essentials.  Chapter 10; Diabetic retinopathy.  Thieme Medical Publishers, Inc, 1999

24. Cugati S, Wang JJ, Rochtchina E, et al. Ten year incidence of retinal vein occlusion in an older population: the Blue Mountains Eye Study.  Arch Opthalmol.  2006;124:726-732

25. Central Vein Occlusion Study Group, Baseline, and early history report.  Arch Ophthalmol. 1993;111(8):1087-1095

26. Ria N. Retinal vein occlusion:pathophysiology and treatment options, Clinical Ophthalmology 2010:4;809-816

27. The Eye Disease Case-Control Study Group.  Risk factors for central retinal vein occlusion. Arch Ophthalmol.  1996;114:545-554

28. American Macular Degeneration Foundation, www.macular.org, accessed 8/15/10

29. The AREDS Research Group, Arch Ophthalmol.  2009;127(9):1168-1174

30. Pauleikhoff D, Barondes MJ, Minassian D, et al. Drusen as risk factors in age-related macular disease.  Am J Ophthalmol 1990;109:38-43

31. Fung AE, Lalwani GA, Rosenfeld PJ, et al.  An optical coherence tomography-guided, variable dosing regimen with intravitreal ranibizumab for neovascular age-related macular degeneration.  Am J Ophthalmol 2007;143:566-83

32. Krebs I, Ansari-Shahrezaei S, Goll A, Binder S. Activity of neovascular lesions treated with bevacizumab: comparison between optical coherence tomography and fluorescein angiography.  Graefes Arch Clin Exp Ophthalmol 2008;246:811-5

33. Regillo CD, Brown GC, Flynn HW.  Vitreoretinal Disease the Essentials.  Chapter 14, Age-Related Macular Degeneration, ppgs. 214-217. Thieme Medical Publishers, Inc, 1999

34. Zweifel S, Spaide R, et al. Ophthalmology, Volume 117, Issue 2; ppgs 303-312, Elsevier Inc, Feb. 2010

35. M Colucciello, Retinal Physician, Sep. 2008, pp 26-32

36. Yannuzzi LA, Negrao S, Iida T, Carvalho C, Rodriguez-Coleman H, Slakter J, Freund KB, Sorenson J, Orlock D, Borodoker N. Retinal angiomatous proliferation in age-related macular degeneration.  Retina 2001; 21(5):416-34.

37. M Colucciello, Retinal Physician, Sep. 2008, pp 26-32

38. Hartnett ME, Weiter JJ, Gardts A, Jalkh AE.  Classification of retinal pigment epithelial detachments associated with drusen.  Graefes Arch Clin Exp Ophthalmol 1992;230:11–19

39. Hartnett ME, Weiter JJ, Staurenghi G, Elsner AE.  Deep retinal vascular anomalous complexes in advanced age-related macular degeneration.  Ophthalmology 1996;103:2042–2053

**40.** Slakter JS, Yannuzzi LA, Schneider U, et al. Retinal choroidal anastomoses and occult choroidal neovascularization in age-related macular degeneration.  Ophthalmology 2000;107:742–754

**41.** Hogan MJ, Alvarado JA, Weddell JE: Histology of the Human Eye.  WB Saunders, Philadelphia, 1971

**42.** R. Margolis, R. Spaide A pilot study of EDI OCT of the choroid in normal eyes, AJO, May, 2009, pg. 811

**43.** Lindblad AS, Clemons TE, Age-Related Eye Disease Study Research Group.  Responsiveness of the National Eye Institute Visual Function Questionnaire to progression to advanced age-related macular degeneration, vision loss and lens opacity.  AREDS Report No. 14. *Arch Ophthalmol.*  2005;123(9):1207-1214

# Retinal Imaging Simplified

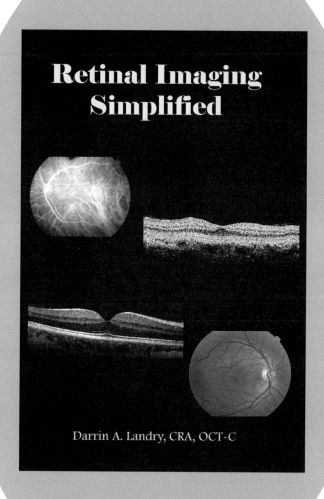

Author Darrin Landry provides a systematic guide of the basics needed to pursue and advance your education in ophthalmic imaging in his first book, *Retinal Imaging Simplified*.

While the majority of ophthalmic photographers have an extensive background in photography, they often require additional training to understand the different imaging modalities, how to properly image the eye, become familiar with retinal pathology, and how to interact with patients.

*Retinal Imaging Simplified* provides the groundwork for improving one's imaging skills while simplifying the process and offers it in an easily accessible, how-to manual, for a seasoned or newly trained photographer, physician, or ophthalmic office personnel.

Get your copy today at

www.brysontaylorpublishing.com

## About the Author

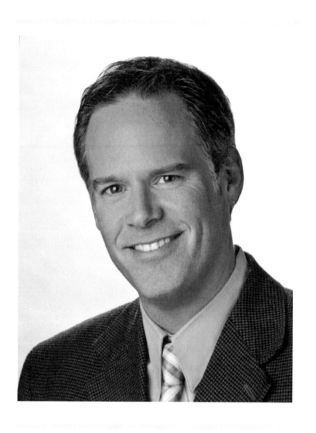

For over 25 years, Mr. Landry has worked in a variety of specialties as a military trained certified surgical technician. In 1989, he became an ophthalmic photographer and technician specializing primarily in retina.

Along with his wife, he is the co-owner of Bryson Taylor Inc., an ophthalmic consulting company started in 1999. As a speaker, consultant, and trainer, Mr. Landry has presented at workshops internationally, is a frequent lecturer for JCAHPO, OPS, ASORN, and the AAO. He is also a consultant for imaging companies, pharmaceutical companies, and medical practices.

He is a Certified Retinal Angiographer and an Optical Coherence Tomographer - Certified, has served as a Subject Matter Expert for the Ophthalmic Photographers' Society Board of Certification, and a past member of the OPS Board of Education.

With numerous awards for his photography and professional speaking engagements, Mr. Landry has been published in various medical journals and textbooks including The Journal of Ophthalmic Photography, Insight, and Viewpoints. He is also the author of *Retinal Imaging Simplified,* a systematic guide to provide the basics to pursue and advance education in ophthalmic imaging.

In his free time, he loves to travel, hike, and spend time with his family. He has made several medical mission trips to Guatemala where he enjoys photographing the native culture.

He currently resides on the coast of Maine with his wife and children.

**www.brysontaylorpublishing.com**

Lightning Source UK Ltd.
Milton Keynes UK
UKRC02n1817300918
329652UK00040B/349